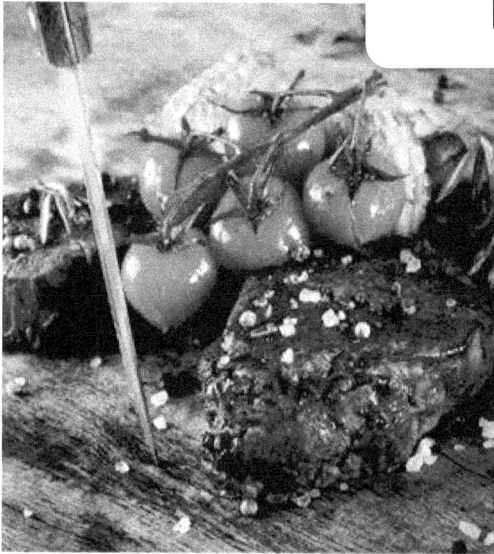

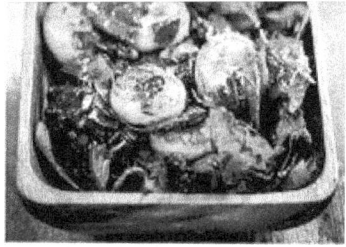

70 ALL-DAY QUALITY RECIPES, 7 DAY STARTER MENU PLAN, STEP-BY-STEP INSTRUCTIONS

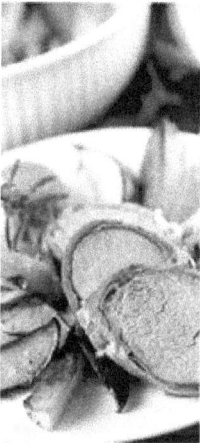

ALL IN 1
PALEO
FOR BEGINNERS

WEIGHT LOSS PROFESSOR

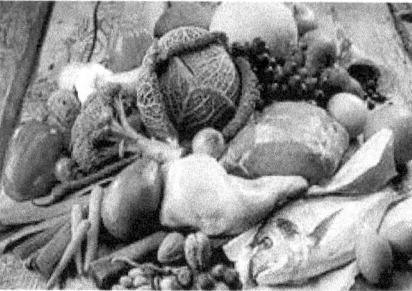

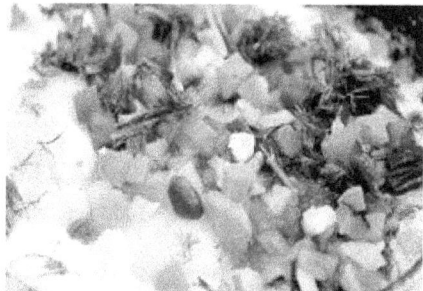

ORLANDO SCOTT

All In 1 Paleo Diet For Beginners

By: Orlando Scott

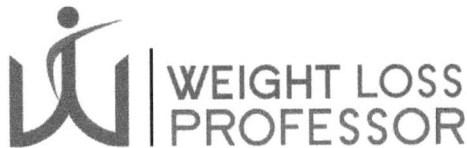

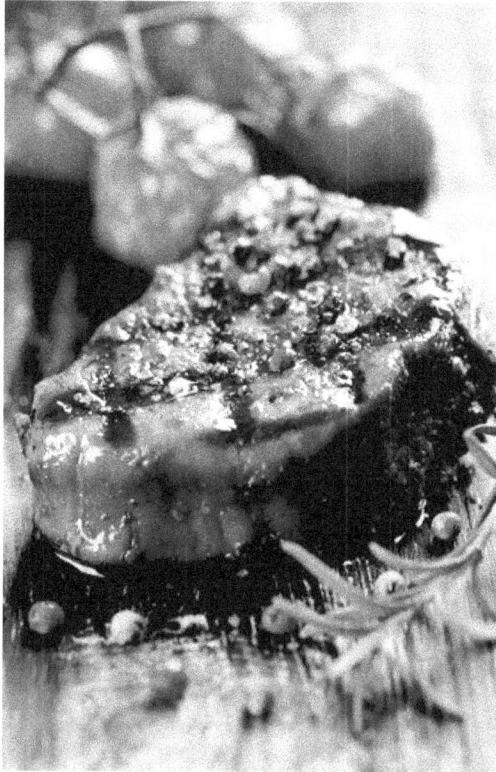

Dear Reader,

Thank You For Purchasing Our Book.

As thanks, we would like to offer a **Free Bonus** exclusive to the first **50 Subscribers** of our mailing list. The link will be available at the end of the book. We will also be providing **lifetime updates** for all subscribers regarding all promotions.

If our book had been useful to you in anyway please remember to leave a **Positive Review** for us on **Amazon.**

Thank you,

Weight Loss Professor

Contents

Disclaimer 8

Introduction 9

Chapter 1: What Is Paleo Diet 11

Chapter 2: Health Benefits of Paleo Diet............... 13

Chapter 3: 7 Day Starter Menu Plan...................... 21

Chapter 4: What to Eat 26

Chapter 5: 70 Paleo Recipes for a Healthier You..... 31

    Coconut Blueberry Oatmeal 31

    Scrambled Eggs with Herbs................................ 33

    Pork Steak with Eggs 34

    Spinach Chorizo Sweet Potato Quiche 35

    Breakfast Burgers 37

    Granny Egg Omelette 39

    Crunchy Citrus Fruit Salad............................... 41

    Burger Salad... 42

    Mexican Beef...44

    Chicken with Tomatoes and Basil 45

    Chicken Lettuce Wraps....................................46

    Thai Coconut Soup.. 47

    Clear Soup Mussels....................................... 49

    Sweet Potato Salad with Bacon and Dill 50

    Marinated Chicken Kebabs............................... 52

Marinated Vegetable Kebabs 54

Sweet Potato Kebabs 57

That's-a some Spicy Meatballs! 59

Grilled Salmon 61

Savory Cashew Stir-fry 63

Paleo Mac and Cheese 65

Directions: 65

Stuffed Bell Peppers 67

Stuffed Tomato Shrimp Salad 69

Green Apple Chicken Salad 70

Sautéed Zucchini Noodles with Shrimp 72

Spaghetti Squash with Ground Beef 74

Mushroom Stew 76

Sausages in Tomato Sauce 78

Frugal Stroganoff 80

"No Beans about It" Pumpkin Chili 82

Pan-Fried Chicken with Steamed Vegetable Medley 84

Leek Casserole 87

Easy Pot Roast 89

Swiss Steak 91

Chicken Artichoke 93

Citrus Chicken Marinade 94

Shrimp Stir-fry 95

Marinated Pork Chops 97

Spiced Pineapple Pork Roast 98

Stuffed Cabbage 100

Glazed Carrots 104

Sautéed Onions.. 105

Roasted Potatoes with Cilantro 106

Butternut Squash Soup.. 107

Gluten Free Tomato Soup....................................... 109

Onion Soup 111

Carrot Soup with Ginger and Zucchini........................... 112

Mushroom Soup 114

Tomato Carrot Soup 116

Summer Zest Soup.. 118

Spicy Almond and Eggplant Soup 120

Lemon Fruit Salad 123

Broccoli Salad with Strawberries 124

Red and Green Salad 125

Waldorf Salad 126

Avocado Shrimp Salad..127

Seasoned Egg Salad 128

Wilted Ginger Spinach.. 129

Sautéed Beet Greens, Version 1 130

Sautéed Beet Greens, Version 2 131

Bitterless Brussel Sprouts....................................... 132

Stewed Apples.. 133

Eggplant and Jicama Stir-fry.................................... 134

Sweet Potato Casserole 136

Beef Bone Broth 138

Avocado and Coconut Milk Salad Dressing 144

Mexican Salsa 145

Cardiovascular Cleanser..146

Sinus and Lymph Tonic 147

Mama's Chock-full Smoothie..148

Golden Milk..149

Chapter 6 - Your Shopping List 151

Chapter 7 - Your Paleo Checklist........................... 155

Conclusion 158

Disclaimer

This eBook has been written for information purposes only. Every effort has been made to make this eBook as complete and accurate as possible. However, there may be mistakes in typography or content. Also, this eBook provides information only up to the publishing date. Therefore, this eBook should be used as a guide and not as the ultimate source.

The purpose of this eBook is to educate. The author and the publisher do not warrant that the information contained in this eBook is fully complete and shall not be responsible for any errors or omissions. The author and publisher shall have neither liability nor responsibility to any person or entity with respect to any loss or damage caused or alleged to be caused directly or indirectly by this eBook.

Introduction

Modern day living forces people to choose on-the-go, easy-to-cook, instant food that lack nutritional value and contains too much fats, sodium, and sugar. Due to this modern-day lifestyle, obesity is on the rise. In 2015, more than one-third (34.9%) of the adult American population is obese. The reason for this is unhealthy eating and lifestyle. The American diet consists of too much calories, too many fats, excessive sodium and too much sugar.

High calorie food such as mayonnaise, French fries, pizza, hotdogs, salami and others can cause fat build up in the body. Calories are needed by the body as it is turned into energy but when you consume too much, your body will store it as fats, which can lead to obesity.

Food rich in trans-fat and saturated fats such as cheeseburgers, potato chips and French fries produce cholesterol in the body, which can lead to heart diseases and cause blockage to your arteries. Sodium-filled food on the other hand causes water retention and raises your blood pressure, which can result to stroke, heart attack and other heart diseases.

Sugar does not only result to tooth decay, it also leads to obesity. Table sugar, fructose, sucrose, molasses and corn syrup provide empty calories that make you crave for more food that is sugary. As a result, your glucose level increases and your risk of becoming overweight is increased. It also increases your risk of having Type II Diabetes wherein glucose builds up in your bloodstream, which results to insulin resistance.

If you want to live a healthier life, you have to make healthy choices when it comes to the food that you eat. The All In 1 Paleo For Beginners book teaches you how to choose healthy food over the unhealthy ones. Some people dislike the idea of going into this diet because they deem it expensive, but that is not the case. This book contains everything you need to know about Paleo Diet as well as numerous Paleo recipes that are low cost, yet tasty and healthy.

Take on the 7-Day Starter Menu Plan using this book as a guide and get ready to be healthier, more energized and happier.

Chapter 1:
What Is Paleo Diet

Paleo Diet has been around for thousands of years. It is based on the diet of the Paleolithic man or the caveman, hence its name. It is consists mainly of fish, meat, fruit and vegetables. Grains, dairy, legumes, and processed food are prohibited.

Since it is based on the Paleolithic diet, it is presumed that the meat you should consume should come from grass-fed, free-range animals. This diet existed way before industrialization, thus, it is based on natural, chemical-free food. Since modern-day living makes it difficult to achieve such criteria, you can choose food that comes closest.

Instead of buying canned berries, choose fresh berries instead. It is better if you can find organic fruits and vegetables. Farmer's markets usually offer fresh produce. Stick to whole, unprocessed foods instead of canned, preserved goods.

To make it easier for you to choose what to eat, refer to the list below:

What to Eat

Fruits

Vegetables

Seafood

Grass-fed Meat

Healthy Fats

Nuts and Seeds

What Not To Eat

Grains

Dairy

Sugars

Processed Foods

Starches

Legumes

Alcohol

As a rule of thumb, stick to food that are whole, raw, and unprocessed. Stay away from GMO food. Always read the labels. If it contains more than three ingredients and you can't even read them, do not take it.

Chapter 2:
Health Benefits of Paleo Diet

It is common knowledge that diet plays a big role in one's health. To live a healthy, happy life, you must learn how to say no to things that can put a threat on your body and health. The Paleo Diet requires you to eat whole, raw, unprocessed food. This means you get to eat healthier, more nutritious food. Therefore, your body gets to enjoy more vitamins, minerals, and nutrients that will keep it nourished and in optimal shape.

The Paleo Diet offers numerous health benefits. To start with, it rids your body of the harmful toxins that have accumulated in your body due to your food and lifestyle choices. Eating fresh, nutritious fruits and vegetables also contains antioxidants that purge toxins out of your body, allowing your body to synthesize nutrients optimally which results to better overall health. When you are disease-free, you get to live a happier life, be able to fulfill your goals and be a more productive member of the society.

In order to get the idea of what benefits a healthier body looks and feels like that are found within the Paleo Diet, let's take a look at the medicinal properties of some herbs, roots and spices that can be added to almost any recipe. Garlic, for example, contains within it a chemical compound called "allicin", derived from hydrogen sulfide, which has multiple health benefits.

Garlic has been found in various studies to support metabolism and boost energy, assist with respiratory issues as well as protect the cardiovascular system. Garlic in conjunction with allisin lowers blood pressure substantially by relaxing the arteries, helping to prevent heart attack and stroke, as well as limiting cancer growth and the progression of several diseases. In order to get these benefits, as well as garlic's powerful antioxidant properties, you have to crush it and allow it to sit for 20 minutes before preparing it in a meal.

Some other common ingredients to begin incorporating into your Paleo Diet on a regular basis are fresh ginger and turmeric. The powder forms of these roots are still effective, turmeric more so than ginger, however you will learn as you continue reading that fresh food is always the best. It is the way our ancestors consumed them, as is the Paleo way, and is the best form of nutrient preservation for ingestion. Both of these roots are highly beneficial to the digestive system for their soothing, inflammation-reducing properties. They also help to balance the pH of the entire body.

The condition of the digestive system, and thus what we choose to put through it, is a key determinant of our overall health. Bloating is significant of inflammation. Stomach and intestinal cramps are signs of dehydration or partially or undigested foods, among other possible causes. Indigestion and acid reflux disease, a.k.a. G.E.R.D., is a sign of anything from a weak valve between the esophagus and the stomach to an overly tight diaphragm that the esophagus runs through, pinching it off and disrupting the natural downward flow of ingested food, to stored stress and anxiety in the body that has accumulated over time through a series of emotionally distressing events. The roots of the causes run deep and consuming fatty or spicy foods only exacerbate the problem.

The Paleo Diet helps to address these issues directly on all levels, starting with the most obvious changes we can make with what we put into our body. By knowing more about how the body works in conjunction with the mind and our mood, we can regulate our systems more positively and live in a higher quality of life.

Is it not common knowledge that if we do not feel good in our body, it is going to be on our mind throughout the day, perhaps even at a subliminal level? And then wouldn't that go to say that the discomfort felt from our body directly affects our attention on what we think about? Going one step further with this logic, if we are feeling poorly in the body that affects us to think poorly, not feeling ourselves and focusing on more negative conditions, our overall mood depreciates too. This cycle can all be reversed by becoming aware of which foods affect us positively and which subtly give us a turn for the worse, no matter how good they *taste*.

Fats, sugar and chemicals from processed foods disrupt the natural flora in your gut, which results to inflammation in your intestinal tract. A blood sugar spike causes your adrenals to produce more cortisol, known as "the stress hormone". Cortisol prevents the production of hydrochloric acid, which your body needs to synthesize food properly. The unprocessed food left in your intestine weakens the gut lining. This can lead to leaky gut syndrome, which means the integrity of your intestinal walls are compromised and the things that are supposed to stay in your digestive tract are leaking out to your bloodstream. This can cause an array of diseases as your immune system will start attacking these leaked particles from your gut and eventually attack its own systems and organs.

Since Paleo Diet recommends eating grass-fed meat, it means you get to consume more lean meat with lesser fats. The reason commercially raised animals are not good for the body is because of the fats that they have accumulated from consuming feeds that are injected with chemicals.

Meat is a good source of protein and protein helps build muscle mass and aids in building new cells. Studies have proven that the more muscles you have, the better your metabolism is. This is because muscles need energy to work. When you have more muscles, your body sends more glycogen to your muscle cells instead of triglycerides to your fat cells. This means you have lesser fats and more lean muscles, making you healthier and more energetic.

Paleo Diet recommends eating more fruits and vegetables and keeping your plate colorful. The color of fruits and vegetables depends on the nutrients and vitamins they offer. Therefore, by making your plate colorful, you get the vitamins and minerals that your body needs. Furthermore, fruits and vegetables are digested easily by the body and they are full of fiber, which also helps in better digestion. Paleo Diet helps keep your digestive system healthy by helping in proper digestion and in getting rid of unwanted toxins in the body.

Paleo for Weight Loss

Paleo Diet requires you to eat raw, unprocessed, whole foods that are rich in vitamins and minerals. Since you are feasting on more fruits and vegetables, lean meat and nuts, your body is undeniably healthier. As your digestive system gets better, nutrients are also transported optimally throughout your body, making your organs work better, which also helps make your immune system stronger.

Sugar, processed and packaged foods that contain corn syrup and the high fructose variety, as well as simple carbohydrates like white grains, pastas, and wheat are all obvious factors that contribute to weight gain. In association with these, leading a relatively inactive lifestyle is another contributor. What may not be obvious is that they go hand in hand.

These ingredients have already been mentioned to cause inflammation in the digestive system. That makes it more difficult to digest food and strains organ function. Inflammation of the stomach not only contributes to leaky gut syndrome, it also builds pressure (along with weight gain) on the diaphragm, which controls lung respiration. Of course, poor breathing habits can stem from a number of different causes although it helps to reduce as many factors as possible, specific food consumption being one of them.

Did you know that medical professionals have directly linked shallow breathing to weight gain and weight retention? The idea has to do with the circulatory system, which is intimately linked with the respiratory system. First of all, shallow breathing does not engage the core where our diaphragm is. This means less muscle use. Secondly, the absence of normal breathing patterns signifies less oxygen to the bloodstream and thus a greater sense of fatigue and inactive tendencies for the affected person. Circulation becomes poor; cells are prevented from receiving necessary nutrients, organ functions slow down, metabolism decreases, metabolic wastes build up that the blood normally removes, and thus the body's processes slowly degrade. Stress builds up in the body, and further stress amounts when the body's environment becomes acidic because of excess sugars.

Stress has not only been proven to raise blood sugars, it has also been linked to weight gain. From a direct habitual standpoint, if a person is used to consoling themselves with food whenever they feel strung out, over time the accumulated stress and eating reaction to that stress will cause them to gain weight. What do people usually reach for with this food consoling habit? That's right: sugary, starchy foods. We don't think about it, we just do it, but it's because sugar consumption temporarily releases endorphins in the brain that give us a kind of high, that is, until the eventual sugar crash. And then we need more.

Furthermore, the eventual breakdown of sugary and starchy foods adds up to more sugar in the bloodstream, causing a spike in blood sugars and then an inevitable drop in energy. This will leave anyone feeling the effects of fatigue shortly after eating along with more hunger pains. The vicious cycle is to crave more of these types of foods to sustain energy levels, and can contribute to a more difficult transition in staying active.

With poor activity habits and an increase in lethargy, the eating habits may continue but the body cannot keep up, and so the unused energy from these sugars get stored as fat within the body. They also, along with other fatty and high cholesterol foods, cause a build-up of plaque in the walls of the veins and arteries, decreasing circulatory flow to the muscles and depriving them of the nutrients and energy that they need to function. All of this spells weight gain, as well as further health complications over time like high blood pressure, high blood pressure, decreased metabolism and a weakened immune system.

These detailed effects are considering that one's diet primarily constitutes the types of food we are talking about to avoid over a long and consistent period of time. They are not intended to scare, rather to help us by being more aware of how we work. The Paleo Diet addresses all of this by removing these foods and their ravaging effects on the body.

By eating more fruits and vegetables and ditching sugar and trans fat, you are helping your body burn fats faster. The body converts fruits and vegetables easily into energy as they contain lesser fats, which results to better metabolism. Faster metabolism means faster and more effective fat burning which translate to weight loss. A note to make here is that no matter what condition you are coming from, whether mild or severe, any state can be reversed into a positive one.

In addition to gaining more energy from eating more fast-acting and energy-sustaining foods that Paleo is synonymous with, you are going to feel more energized to *do* more. Your brain function will improve, and cloud-mindedness will dissipate. It will still take a conscious mental effort to develop consistency and firmly establish better, healthier habits. However, you will now have the support and reserves to not only have a stronger motivation for exercise and activity, you will be provided with a consistent source of energy to engage in it without feeling physically drained.

Therefore, you can increase your effort in losing weight with the Paleo diet substantially by working with the physical benefits it is already providing you. Use them to mentally carry you through into a self-supportive attitude that encourages you to do more. Start by congratulating yourself every time you eat and stick with the Paleo Diet, knowing that this is going to help you turn your life around. It can do as much for you as you allow it to, and from there it depends how far you choose to run with it.

See this diet as your ticket to doing things you had aspired to but didn't feel you could before. Take up an aerobics class, clean the cobwebs off your bike and go out for a ride, or call up a friend and go explore a hiking trail. You can share with them how great the Paleo Diet makes you feel in your body and your mind, just by shuffling up your meal ingredients a bit.

The great thing about it is that you can still indulge your taste buds in rich, flavorful foods and recipes. Their preference might take some adjusting but that is just the sugar addiction talking that will eventually disappear. Trust that it is an addiction, too. Biologically as well as psychologically speaking, the addictive effects of sugar on the body have been compared to those of cocaine. Remember that sugars play upon the endorphin levels in a big way. With the Paleo switch, the rest of your body will be thanking you immediately, and it will show its gratitude through stabilizing and improving mood levels as well as the subsequent evidence of weight loss.

The key to losing weight effectively in Paleo is by eating just enough fats, more vegetables, lean meats and eggs. You can still snack on fruits and nuts but you should keep it to a minimum. You can have two fruits in a day and a palm full of nuts for snacks.

You do not need to count the calories in each of your meals. That only adds to the stress and frustration of staying on a diet. This is what makes Paleo a better and effective choice. You don't even have to eat on proportions. You eat when your body tells you to eat. You alone know how your body works, listen to it, and follow it. Just remember to focus on eating more vegetables and lean meats. To make it easier, make it 70% vegetables (raw or cooked), 20% lean meats, and 10% fruits and nuts. This means your plate should be full of vegetables with a serving of meat and a piece of fruit.

Chapter 3:
7 Day Starter Menu Plan

This Paleo sample menu will help guide you through your Paleo Diet. You can adjust it according to your needs.

Day 1

Breakfast

Stir fried vegetables in coconut oil with one boiled egg.

One crunchy fruit such as apple, pear, persimmon, etc.

Lunch

Chicken Salad with lots of green leafy vegetables and a handful of nuts.

Dinner

Burger Patties made from lean meat and fried in butter.

Vegetable Salad

Salsa

Day 2

Breakfast

Egg frittata with avocados

A piece of fruit

Lunch

Stir-fried vegetables in coconut oil with lean beef strips

Dinner

Salmon fried in butter

Vegetable salad

Day 3

Breakfast

Devilled eggs with mashed potato filling

One fruit

Lunch

Roasted chicken with asparagus

Vegetable Salad

Dinner

Stir fried ground lean beef with vegetables

Berries

Day 4

Breakfast

Egg omelet in olive oil with vegetables

Some Berries

Lunch

Poached chicken salad with seasonal vegetables tossed in olive oil

Vegetable Salad with nuts

Dinner

Lean pork steak with potatoes and veggies

One fruit

Day 5

Breakfast

Boiled egg

Breakfast casserole with turkey sausages and sweet potatoes

Lunch

Chicken sandwich with lettuce leaves and vegetables

Berries

Dinner

Grilled chicken with vegetables

Salsa

Day 6

Breakfast

Sautéed Vegetables with thin lean pork slices

A fruit

Lunch

Steamed chicken breast sandwich with lettuce leaves and vegetables

Some berries

Dinner

Baked broccoli with egg

Day 7

Breakfast

Mixed bean salad with olive oil dressing

Citrus Salad with vinaigrette

A fruit

Lunch

Fried pork in coconut oil with vegetables

Dinner

Baked salmon with butter and vegetables

Berries

There is no need to watch your calories with this diet, but if you are trying to lose weight, limit your intake of carbohydrates, potatoes, and nuts.

Chapter 4:
What to Eat

Not all foods are allowed in the Paleo Diet. For an easy reference, check the list below:

Allowed Foods

Grass-fed meats/Free-range animals

- Cow

- Chicken

- Goat

- Sheep

- Turkey

- Pig

Sea-caught fish/ seafood

- Salmon

- Mackerel

- Tuna

- Shrimp

- Lobster

- Clams

- Sardines

Organic fresh fruits

- Avocado
- Apple
- Banana
- Blackberries
- Blueberries
- Cantaloupe
- Figs
- Grapes
- Guava
- Oranges
- Peaches
- Papaya
- Plums
- Raspberries
- Tangerine
- Lemon
- Lime
- Lychee

- Mango
- Pineapple
- Strawberries

Organic fresh vegetables

- Avocado
- Asparagus
- Artichoke
- Brussel Sprouts
- Broccoli
- Spinach
- Cabbage
- Carrots
- Celery
- Cauliflower
- Eggplant
- Green Onions
- Parsley
- Zucchini

If you are into weight loss, limit your intake of these vegetables as they are starchy.

- Acorn Squash

- Beets

- Butternut Squash

- Potato

- Sweet Potato

- Yam

Healthy Fats

- Avocado Oil

- Coconut Oil

- Macadamia Oil

- Olive Oil

- Grass-fed Butter

Nuts

- Almonds

- Pecans

- Pumpkin Seeds

- Pine Nuts

- Cashew

- Hazelnuts

- Sunflower Seeds

- Walnuts

- Macadamia Nuts

Chapter 5:
70 Paleo Recipes for a Healthier You

To help you get started with paleo, here are low cost recipes you can try.

Breakfast

Coconut Blueberry Oatmeal

Ingredients:

1 cup	Full Fat Coconut Milk
2	Ripe Bananas, peeled and cut into small cubes
¼ cup	Coconut Butter
1 teaspoon	Vanilla Extract
1 tablespoon	Gelatin
1 cup	Fresh Blueberries
1 ½ cup	Coconut Meat, shredded finely

Directions:

1. Heat pot on a stove over medium temperature.

2. Pour in coconut milk, coconut butter, vanilla extract, banana and a pinch of salt. Mix and bring to a boil.

3. Lower down heat and simmer for 10 minutes while stirring from time to time to break down banana pieces.

4. Stir in gelatin and mix until well dissolved.

5. Mix in blueberries and simmer for another 2 minutes.

6. Turn off heat and add shredded coconuts.

7. Let sit for a few minutes to soften coconut meat.

Scrambled Eggs with Herbs

Ingredients:

2 tablespoons	Ghee or Butter
5 medium	Eggs, beaten
½ cup	Goat Cheese, crumbled
½ teaspoon	Garlic Powder
½ teaspoon	Dried Basil
1 teaspoon	Dried Dill
1/8 cup	Raw Walnuts, chopped
1 pinch	Salt
1 pinch	Ground Pepper

Directions:

1. Heat ghee or butter in a skillet over medium heat.

2. Stir in beaten eggs.

3. Add dill, garlic powder, basil, pepper and salt.

4. When eggs are almost done, turn off heat and add goat cheese.

5. Serve with chopped walnuts on top.

Pork Steak with Eggs

Ingredients:

1 large	Lean Pork Steak
3 tablespoons	Tallow, ghee or butter
2 medium	Eggs
1 pinch	Paprika
1 pinch	Salt
1 pinch	Pepper

Directions:

1. Leave your steak standing on room temperature for 40 minutes before cooking to make it juicy and easier to cook.

2. Melt fats in pan over medium heat.

3. Season steak with salt, pepper and paprika. Add into the pan and cook each side until golden brown or depending on your taste.

4. Set aside in serving plate.

5. In the same pan, crack open egg and season with salt, paprika and pepper. Cook to your liking. Do the same with the other egg.

6. Serve with steak on the side.

Spinach Chorizo Sweet Potato Quiche

Ingredients:

4 large	Sweet Potatoes, cut into very thin rounds
5 large	Eggs, beaten
2 cups	Fresh Spinach
3 slices	Bacon, cooked and crumbled
1	Onion, sliced
1 clove	Garlic, minced
2 tablespoons	Fresh Chives
2 tablespoons	Olive Oil
2 tablespoons	Ghee, Lard or Butter
1 pinch	Salt
1 pinch	Ground Pepper

Directions:

1. Preheat your oven to 400°F.

2. Arrange thin potato rounds into circular pattern in a pie dish. This will serve as the crust for the quiche. Drizzle with olive oil, salt and pepper.

3. Cook in the oven for 15 to 20 minutes.

4. While doing so, melt ghee, butter or lard in a skillet over medium heat and sauté garlic and onion.

5. Stir in spinach and cook until wilted. Set aside.

6. When sweet potatoes are fork tender, reduce oven heat to 375°F.

7. In a bowl, combine beaten eggs, sautéed spinach, chives and bacon. Pour mixture into the potato crust and cook in the oven for 30 to 35 minutes or until eggs are well set.

Breakfast Burgers

Ingredients:

5 to 6 ounces	Ground beef
2	Eggs
½ cup	Onion, chopped
1 cup	Fresh spinach leaves
½ cup	Tomato, diced or chopped into long, thin pieces
2 tablespoons	Coconut oil
1 tablespoon	Coconut aminos
1 ½ teaspoons	Worcestershire sauce
A pinch	Salt
A dash	Pepper
A dash	Chipotle chili powder
A sprinkling	Turmeric
A dash	Oregano
A pinch	Thyme
A dusting	Cinnamon

Directions:

1. Heat 1 tablespoon of oil in a frying pan on low. Once heated, raise heat to medium or medium-high and add ground beef to brown along with onions.

2. Season beef and onions with liquids and spices while cooking. Add tomatoes in before beef has completely browned.

3. Add 1 more tablespoon of oil and reduce heat to medium-low. Break eggs over beef, keeping yolks intact. When the whites cook to semi-translucence, separate beef with spatula or wooden spoon and mix eggs together with them (yolks may break).

4. Immediately remove pan from heat after step 3 and create a thin layer with the spinach on top. Cover the pan and let sit for 1 minute.

5. Serve right after 1 minute. Spinach will be wilted, eggs will be only partially scrambled, yolks still somewhat runny.

Granny Egg Omelette

Ingredients:

2 large	Farm-Raised Eggs
¼ cup	Onion, chopped
¼ cup	Green Bell Pepper, chopped
¼ cup	Red Bell Pepper, chopped
2 teaspoons	Oil (Olive, Coconut or otherwise)
A pinch	Salt
A dash	Coarse Ground Black Pepper
A dash	Chipotle Chili powder
A sprinkling	Turmeric
A light touch	Cinnamon powder

Directions:

1. In a small bowl, beat the eggs well until they are frothy with lots of little bubbles. The key to a fluffy omelet is not adding milk, but beating them long enough to trap air inside. Once this is done, add the spices into the eggs and beat them a little bit more to mix. Set aside.

2. You will need a small frying pan, around 6" in diameter and a lid that seals well with it. Heat 1 teaspoon of oil in the pan on low heat, coating the surface completely, including the sides. Add in the onions and cook on

medium-high heat, stirring occasionally until they become translucent and slightly caramelized. Add in the peppers halfway and keep stirring every so often.

3. Add the second teaspoon of oil into the pan and disperse it evenly. Beat the eggs well once more, as some of the spices will have settled to the bottom. After 15 to 30 seconds of beating them, immediately pour the eggs into the pan with the vegetables, making sure that they are coated evenly. Scrape as much of the eggs and spices from the bowl into the pan as you can.

4. Cover the pan, reduce to medium-low heat and cook for about 4 to 5 minutes. Check on the omelet to see that the middle is no longer liquid or runny. That is when you know it is done.

5. Remove from heat. Use a knife or metal spatula and run it along the edge of the pan, then gently use the spatula to get underneath the omelet and remove it from the pan. It should look like a delicious egg pancake. Enjoy.

Crunchy Citrus Fruit Salad

Ingredients:

4 medium	Green apples, cored and diced
2 large	Pears, cored and diced
1 stalk	Celery, diced
2 cups	Seedless Green Grapes, halved
½ teaspoon	Cinnamon
½ cup	Juice from freshly squeezed orange
½ fruit	Lemon, juiced
¼ cup	Pine Nuts
2 tablespoons	Olive Oil

Directions:

1. In a deep bowl, mix together lemon juice, orange juice, olive oil and cinnamon.

2. In a separate salad bowl, combine all fruits. Top with dressing and toss until everything is well coated.

3. Refrigerate for a few minutes and serve cold.

Lunch

Burger Salad

Ingredients:

1 ½ lb	Ground Beef
1 head	Romaine Lettuce, torn to pieces
1 medium	Red Onion, julienned
1 small	Avocado, diced, peeled and deseeded
3 small	Tomatoes, diced
4	Dill Pickles, halved
½ cup	Barbecue Sauce
1 ½ tablespoon	Yellow Mustard
1 ½ tablespoon	Dijon Mustard

Directions:

1. Brown ground beef in a skillet over medium heat. Remove excess fat.

2. Turn off heat and stir in mustards and BBQ sauce. Mix until beef is well coated and set aside.

3. Divide torn lettuce leaves in individual serving plates and top with beef mixture.

4. Add tomatoes, avocados, onions and pickles (two halves each serving).

Mexican Beef

Ingredients:

½ cup	Ground Beef
1 small	Onion
1 medium	Green Bell Pepper
1 medium	Red Bell Pepper
1 pinch	Salt
1 pinch	Ground Black Pepper
¼ cup	Salsa
1 large	Egg

Directions:

1. Sauté onions and pepper in a frying pan over medium heat until tender.

2. Stir in ground beef and season with salt and pepper.

3. Cook until ground beef is completely brown. Add salsa.

4. Mix until ground beef is evenly coated with salsa. Transfer to a serving plate and set aside.

5. In the same frying pan, fry egg according to your taste. Season with salt and pepper.

6. Top sautéed ground beef with fried egg.

Chicken with Tomatoes and Basil

Ingredients:

4	Chicken Breasts, skinned and sliced thinly
2 tablespoons	Ghee or Butter
1 cup	Cherry Tomatoes, halved
4 large	Basil Leaves, chopped coarsely
2 cloves	Garlic, minced

Directions:

1. Heat ghee or butter in a pan over medium heat and sauté tomatoes until soft and skin is starting to peel off from the pulp.

2. Add chicken and mix to make sure it's coated with the liquid from the tomatoes.

3. Season with salt and pepper. Make sure the chicken is cooked through and through.

4. When chicken is already brown on all sides, mix in garlic and basil.

5. Cook for 1 more minute and remove from heat. Serve.

Chicken Lettuce Wraps

Ingredients:

½ lb	Chicken Breast, sliced into small pieces
1 teaspoon	Fish Sauce
2 tablespoons	Coconut Aminos or Tamari
1	Onion, diced
1 clove	Garlic, diced
2 tablespoons	Butter or Coconut Oil
1 tablespoon	Salsa, plus more for toppings

Directions:

1. Heat butter or oil in a pan over medium heat and sauté onions.

2. Stir in chicken and cook until tender.

3. Season with coconut aminos or tamari. Mix in fish sauce and salsa until mixture is thick.

4. Add garlic and toss.

5. Turn off heat and serve on lettuce wraps. Top with more salsa.

Thai Coconut Soup

Ingredients:

1 lb	Boneless skinless chicken breasts, cubed OR Shrimp, peeled, rinsed and deveined
1 bunch	Scallions (Green onion), chopped and sliced to 1" strips
½ cup	Red Bell Pepper, sliced
½ cup	Green Bell pepper, sliced
4 cloves	Garlic, peeled and minced
3 ounces	Fresh ginger, peeled and grated
1 cup	Mushrooms (Shiitake, Baby Bella or your choice), chopped into large chunks
4 cups	Water or chicken broth
1 ½ tablespoons	Fish sauce
2 teaspoons	Red curry paste
1 small	Lime, juiced
2 tablespoons	Butter, Ghee, or desired Oil
14 ounces	Coconut milk
1/3 cup	Cilantro, coarsely chopped
½ teaspoon	Salt

½ teaspoon   Coarse Ground Black Pepper

Directions:

1. In a large pot over medium heat, heat the butter, ghee or whichever fat you have chosen to use.

2. Sauté the scallions, ginger and garlic at a constant stir until tender, roughly 5 minutes.

3. Stir in the prepared red and green peppers, mushrooms, and red curry paste, cooking for about 3 minutes.

4. Add the water or chicken broth to the pot, along with coconut milk, fish sauce, and chicken or shrimp. (Note, if using shrimp, do not add to soup until last 10 minutes of cooking)

5. Bring to a boil, reduce to a simmer and cook 15 to 20 minutes.

6. Stir in cilantro, seasonings and lime juice.

7. Immediately remove from heat and serve in bowls at desired portions.

Clear Soup Mussels

Ingredients:

2 lbs	Fresh Mussels
2 cups	Water
5 cloves	Garlic, minced
2	Onions, chopped
1 inch	Ginger, crushed
1 bunch	Lemongrass
3 tablespoons	Ghee or Butter
2 tablespoons	Fish Sauce
½ teaspoon	Salt
½ teaspoon	Ground Black Pepper

Directions:

1. In a large pot, melt butter or ghee over medium temperature.

2. Sauté garlic, onions and ginger.

3. Pour in water and allow to boil.

4. Add mussels. Mix in fish sauce, salt and pepper.

5. Reduce heat to low and simmer until mussels are cooked thoroughly.

Sweet Potato Salad with Bacon and Dill

Ingredients:

4 medium	Sweet Potatoes, peeled and cut into cubes
10 slices	Bacon
6 cloves	Garlic, minced
4 tablespoons	Fresh Dill, chopped finely
4 tablespoons	Juice from freshly squeezed lime
3 tablespoons	Olive Oil
1 tablespoon	Balsamic Vinegar
2	Scallions, chopped for garnish
	Pumpkin Seeds/Sunflower Seeds for garnish

Directions:

1. Preheat oven to 350 °F.

2. Line baking sheet with foil and arrange bacon slices. Bake until crispy. Set aside.

3. Reserve bacon fats for later.

4. In a large roasting pan, combine bacon fats, sweet potatoes and garlic. Transfer into the same baking sheet

you used for the bacon and roast in the middle rack of the oven until they start to caramelize. Stir occasionally.

5. While at it, whisk olive oil, lime juice, balsamic vinegar and dill. Set aside.

6. Transfer roasted sweet potatoes in a serving bowl and crumble bacon on top of it. Drizzle with dill-lime dressing. Toss to coat evenly. Garnish with pumpkin seeds/sunflower seeds and chopped scallions.

Marinated Chicken Kebabs

Ingredients:

22 – 28 ounces	Whole Chicken Breast, trimmed and cut into 1" cubes
8	Limes, juiced
¼ cup	Cilantro, finely chopped
1 ½ tablespoons	Olive Oil
½ teaspoon	Red Pepper Flakes
1/8 teaspoon	Salt
3	Cloves of Garlic, peeled and minced.
4 –	8Skewers (Metal or Wooden, however if they are wooden then soak them in water overnight so that they do not burn when grilling)

Directions:

1. Add ingredients together in a measuring cup or container that can pour easily without spilling. Mix well.

2. In a large plastic bag, add chicken and then pour marinade mixture in. Seal the bag and shake vigorously, making sure everything is well coated.

3. Put bag in refrigerator for 2 – 3 hours, but not any longer than that! Any longer and the marinade will begin to toughen the chicken meat.

4. Remove the bag from the refrigerator and skew the chicken with the skewers in desired quantities, leaving at least 1" of space on each end of the skewer. Place the skewers on a baking sheet to bring to the grill. Pour the marinade into a bowl and grab a basting brush.

5. Grill the skewered chicken until browned or slightly blackened. Rotate the skewers occasionally to cook all sides evenly. While grilling, use the brush to occasionally baste the chicken.

6. When finished grilling, place the skewers back onto the baking sheet and bring to a plate where you may remove the chicken from the skewers. Serve while hot!

Marinated Vegetable Kebabs

Ingredients:

1 large	Red Bell Pepper, cut into large pieces (about ¾" to 1")
1 large	Green Bell Pepper, cut into large pieces (about ¾" to 1")
1 large	Red Onion, cut into chunks so the layers stay together (same size as the bell peppers)
3 – 5 ounces	Baby Bella or White Mushrooms, cut into thick pieces
1 large	Green Zucchini, cut into large, thick pieces
1 large	Yellow Squash, cut into large, thick pieces
2 tablespoons	Olive Oil
1 cup	Red Wine Vinegar
1 cup	Balsamic Vinegar
3	Cloves of Garlic, peeled and minced
1 ½ teaspoons	Oregano
1 ½ teaspoons	Basil
½ teaspoon	Salt

¾ teaspoon	Coarse Ground Black Pepper
8 – 12	Skewers (Metal or Wooden, however if they are wooden then soak them in water overnight so that they do not burn when grilling)

Directions:

1. Combine the olive oil, vinegars, garlic and spices together and mix well in a container that pours easily, or a large bowl if there is enough space in your refrigerator.

2. Pour the marinade into a large plastic bag or keep in a bowl and add the veggies to it, mixing them carefully to make sure that they are fully coated without separating the onions.

3. Place the sealed bag or covered bowl in the refrigerator to marinade overnight.

4. Remove the marinated vegetables from the refrigerator and skewer them. Create an even variety on each skewer by alternating the vegetables. Leave at least an inch of space on both ends of the skewers and place them on a baking sheet when finished.

5. Bring the remaining marinade, a basting brush, and the skewers out to the grill. Grill the vegetable kebabs, rotating them occasionally so they cook evenly until they are slightly withered and/or blackened. While grilling, baste the vegetables with the remaining marinade.

6. When done grilling, set the skewers back onto the tray and remove the vegetables from them onto a plate. Serve and praise the grill gods!

Sweet Potato Kebabs

Ingredients:

3 medium	Sweet Potatoes, cut into large, 1" cubes
3 tablespoons	Coconut Oil
½ teaspoon	Cinnamon powder
½ teaspoon	Ground Nutmeg
4 – 6	Skewers (Metal or Wooden, however if they are wooden then soak them in water overnight so that they do not burn when grilling)

Directions:

1. Preheat the oven to 400° Fahrenheit.

2. Heat the coconut oil in a saucepan on low until it turns to a liquid.

3. Add the cinnamon and nutmeg to the coconut oil, stirring until it is mixed well.

4. In a bowl, add the sweet potatoes and pour the coconut oil marinade over them, mixing until they are completely coated.

5. Put the sweet potatoes on a baking sheet and into the oven. Half-bake them for 20 to 25 minutes.

6. Remove the sweet potatoes from the oven and skewer them, making sure to leave at least 1" of space at both ends of the skewers. Place the skewers on a baking sheet and bring them out to the grill.

7. Grill the sweet potatoes until browned or slightly blackened, rotating the skewers occasionally so that the sweet potatoes are cooked evenly on all sides. It should not take much time, about 5 – 7 minutes.

8. Remove the skewers from the grill onto the baking sheet, and then remove the sweet potatoes from the skewers onto a plate.

9. Serve hot!

That's-a some Spicy Meatballs!

Meatball Ingredients:

1 cup	Flaxseed Meal
2 1/2 lb	Ground Beef, Pork and Veal, mixed together
1/4 cup	Onion, chopped
2	Eggs, slightly beaten
1/2 teaspoon	Salt
1/4 teaspoon	Pepper

Meatball Directions:

1. Preheat the oven to 400° Fahrenheit

2. Combine above ingredients thoroughly in a large bowl.

3. Shape into meatballs of the size that you desire, or 1 1/2 inches in diameter.

4. Place onto an ungreased baking sheet and bake in the oven for 15 minutes, turning once until brown.

Spicy Sauce Ingredients:

15 ounces	Tomato Sauce
¼ cup	Organic Ketchup
¼ cup	Onion, chopped

¼ cup	Pickle Relish
¼ teaspoon	Organic Honey or Agave sweetener
¼ teaspoon	Coarse Ground Black Pepper
½ teaspoon	Crushed Red Pepper Flakes
2 tablespoons	Worcestershire Sauce
2 tablespoons	White Vinegar

Spicy Sauce Directions:

1. In a large saucepan on low heat, combine all the ingredients, mixing well, and simmer for 1 hour, stirring occasionally.

2. Add the meatballs and keep hot

3. Serve with any vegetable pasta dish of your healthy heart's desire.

Grilled Salmon

Ingredients:

8 ounces	Wild Caught Salmon (Sockeye, Scottish, etc.)
1 ½ tablespoons	Dijon Mustard
1 tablespoon	Balsamic Vinegar
¼ teaspoon	Lemon Pepper
¼ teaspoon	Garlic Salt
1 ½ tablespoons	Organic Honey

Directions:

1. Preheat the oven to 400° Fahrenheit.

2. Combine all of the ingredients except for the salmon in a medium-sized bowl.

3. Lightly oil a baking sheet or lay a sheet of aluminum foil over it to prevent the salmon from sticking, and then place the salmon on the baking sheet.

4. Spread the seasoning over the top of the salmon evenly

5. Place in the oven and bake until you see the white fat of the fish thoroughly rise to the surface. You can also use the fork test by sticking a fork in the fish and twisting it. When the meat flakes off easily, you know it is done cooking; about 8 minutes if thawed and 12 if minutes frozen.

6. ON THE OTHER HAND, if you choose to grill it you can skip step 1 and place the seasoned salmon directly on the grill to cook for about 5 minutes or less, using the fork or fat test to assure that it is cooked thoroughly.

Savory Cashew Stir-fry

Ingredients:

¾ cup	Yellow Squash, sliced
¾ cup	Green Zucchini, sliced
1 ¼ cups	Eggplant, chopped
7 small to medium	Brussel Sprouts, cut into quarters
1 ¼ cups	Red Onion, diced
1 cup	Carrots, sliced
¾ cup	Red Bell Pepper, chopped
¾ cup	Green Bell Pepper, chopped
1 ½ cups	Kale, shredded
1 ½ cups	Fresh Spinach leaves
½ cup	Cashew halves and pieces
½ ounce	Fresh Ginger, peeled and minced
3	Cloves of Garlic, peeled and minced
¼ teaspoon	Cinnamon powder
½ teaspoon	Chipotle Chili powder
½ teaspoon	Coarse Ground Black Pepper
¼ teaspoon	Turmeric

| ¼ teaspoon | Salt |
| 2 ½ tablespoons | Coconut Oil |

Directions:

1. In a large frying pan or wok on low heat, cook coconut oil until melted and cover the surface of the pan including the sides. Add in the ginger and garlic, cooking and stirring for 1 minute.

2. Add in the brussel sprouts, eggplant and carrots, stirring them until completely coated. These go in first because they will take longer to soften. Cover and cook for an additional 2 to 3 minutes.

3. Increase to medium-low heat. Combine the rest of the vegetables except the kale and spinach, mixing them well until all vegetables are coated.

4. Add in the spices and cashews. Mix well to coat all vegetables so the spices are dispersed evenly. Cover again and cook for about 7 to 10 minutes until the brussel sprouts are tender.

5. Return to low heat and add kale and spinach leaves on top. Cover once more and cook for an additional 2 to 3 minutes.

6. Remove from heat. Stir and mix kale and spinach leaves in with the rest of the vegetables. Cover and let cool for up to 5 minutes.

7. Serve. Makes 6 servings.

Paleo Mac and Cheese

Ingredients:

1 head	Cauliflower, grated with medium-sized holes OR chopped to desired bite-sized pieces
2 cloves	Garlic, peeled and grated (using perforated side of grater)
1/3 cup	Onion, finely chopped
3 tablespoons	Almond, Tapioca, or other flour
2 cups	Coconut, almond or flax milk
5 tablespoons	nutritional yeast
3 tablespoons	Olive (or other) oil
3 teaspoons	Tomato sauce
¼ teaspoon	apple cider vinegar
Up to ¼ teaspoon	Turmeric
2 to 3 tablespoons	Butter or Ghee for a creamier sauce (optional)
A pinch	Salt

Directions:

1. Steam the prepared cauliflower, 3 to 4 minutes.

2. While steaming cauliflower, heat oil in a pot over medium-low heat and combine all other ingredients in

pot except the flour and butter or ghee. Simmer, stirring constantly.

3. Create a rue by combining 3 tablespoons of cheese sauce to 1 tablespoon of desired flour. Whisk rue back into cheese sauce until it thickens. Repeat this process as needed until acquiring desired thickness.

4. Place desired portion of cauliflower in serving bowl(s), covering with cheese sauce and mix together.

Stuffed Bell Peppers

Ingredients:

4 large	Bell peppers, any color with the tops cut off horizontally
1 lb	Ground beef
1 large	Cauliflower head, quartered
1 cup	Tomato sauce
2 stalks	Celery, chopped
½ large	Onion, chopped
1/3 cup	Scallions or chives
1 teaspoon	Basil
1 teaspoon	Oregano
¾ teaspoon	Thyme
½ teaspoon	Coarse Ground Black Pepper
½ teaspoon	Salt
1 tablespoon	Olive oil

Directions:

1. Use a cheese grater with medium-sized holes to grate the cauliflower sections into Paleo-friendly rice-sized bits. Set aside.

2. Add olive oil to frying pan over medium to medium-high heat. Fry ground beef until just browning along with onions and celery.

3. Reduce to low heat and add cauliflower rice, cooking together for a few minutes. Taste cauliflower rice to desired tenderness, add water by the tablespoon for longer cooking time if necessary.

4. Preheat oven to 375° Fahrenheit.

5. Remove beef and rice mixture from heat and place into a medium bowl. Add spices and mix all these ingredients together.

6. Spoon mixture into bell peppers then drizzle the tomato sauce on top.

7. Be sure to cut the seedy stems off the bell pepper tops. Cover the bell peppers with the tops and place them on a baking sheet or in a glass baking dish. Place in the oven for 30 to 40 minutes until peppers are slightly roasted.

8. Remove from oven and remove tops, serving as a garnish on the side. Add chives on top as a garnish. Make 4 servings.

Stuffed Tomato Shrimp Salad

Ingredients:

1 lb	Large shrimp; cooked, shelled, deveined, and left cold
3 large	Tomatoes (Beefsteak variety)
1 cup	Celery, diced
½ cup	Onion, finely chopped
¾ cup	Mayonnaise
A sprinkle	Salt
A sprinkle	Coarse Ground Black Pepper

Directions:

1. Remove tails from shrimp and cut into 4 to 5 pieces each.

2. In a medium to large-sized bowl, combine shrimp with the other ingredients except the tomatoes.

3. Cut each tomato in half vertically, scoop out the insides (flesh and seeds) and discard or use for another recipe.

4. Spoon the shrimp mixture into each tomato and serve cold or at room temperature.

Green Apple Chicken Salad

Ingredients:

2 to 4	Boneless, skinless chicken breasts
1 cup	Water or chicken broth
6 tablespoons	Olive oil
A pinch	Salt
A dash	Coarse Ground Black Pepper
A dusting	Paprika
2 cups	Romaine lettuce
2 cups	Kale
2 stalks	Scallions (green onions, or onion of your choice), chopped into small pieces.
1 large	Tomato, diced
1 medium	Red bell pepper, chopped
1 medium	Green bell pepper, chopped
1 medium	Cucumber, sliced or diced
1 medium	Granny Smith apple

Directions:

1. Heat the olive oil in a fry pan over medium to medium-high heat.

2. Add the chicken breasts, sprinkling the spices on top of each side. Brown each side of the breasts to sear in the juices.

3. Pour in the water or chicken broth, turn the heat down to a simmer and cover the pan for 25 to 30 minutes until thoroughly cooked or when meat thermometer reaches 165° Fahrenheit.

4. While the chicken is cooking, prepare and combine the salad ingredients in a large bowl.

5. Cut and cube the warm chicken and add to the salad. Portion into serving sizes. Top with avocado dressing found in the Accessory Recipes section.

Dinner

Sautéed Zucchini Noodles with Shrimp

Ingredients:

4 medium	Zucchini, use spiralizer to make it noodles
2 tablespoons	Coconut Oil
6 cloves	Garlic, minced
6 cups	Grape Tomatoes, halved
24 pcs	Pre-cooked Shrimps, tails removed
1 sprig	Fresh Basil, chopped
1 pinch	Salt
1 pinch	Pepper

Directions:

1. Use spiralizer to turn zucchini into noodles and set aside.

2. Set large skillet into medium temperature and heat coconut oil.

3. Sauté garlic until soft and aromatic.

4. Adjust heat to low and stir in shrimps. Add tomatoes and cook until soft.

5. Mix in zucchini noodles. Add basil, salt and pepper. Cook zucchini until soft while stirring from time to time.

6. You may top with goat cheese, mozzarella or feta if you want.

7. Garnish with freshly chopped basil.

Spaghetti Squash with Ground Beef

Ingredients:

1 ½ lbs	*Ground Beef*
1 ½ cups	*Beef Stock or Water*
2	*Onions, diced*
1 can (29oz)	*Tomato Sauce*
1 can (29oz)	*Diced Tomatoes*
4 cloves	*Garlic, diced*
3 pieces	*Bay leaves*
1 tablespoon	Italian Seasoning
1 tablespoon	Coconut Aminos (soy sauce)
1 tablespoon	Seasoned Salt
1 teaspoon	Pepper
1 teaspoon	Garlic Powder
1 medium	Spaghetti Squash

Directions:

1. In a large pot or Dutch oven, sauté ground meat over medium heat until brown.

2. Stir in onions and sauté until tender.

3. Pour in beef stock or water, tomatoes, tomato sauce, Italian seasoning, garlic, bay leaves, seasoned salt,

coconut aminos, pepper and garlic powder. Mix well and cover. Lower heat to low and cook for 20 minutes.

4. Stir and increase heat to medium. Simmer for 15 minutes.

5. Turn off heat and cool until warm enough to touch.

6. Stir in cooked spaghetti squash and serve.

Mushroom Stew

Ingredients:

1 ½ lbs	Brown mushrooms (Baby Bella, Portobello, shiitake, or others), rinsed and sliced
½ pound	Wild mushrooms (Oyster, etc.), rinsed and sliced
3 tablespoons	Sesame, olive oil or other
1 large	Red onion, julienned
3 small	Tomatoes, chopped
1 tablespoon	Tomato paste
3 cloves	Garlic, peeled and minced
1 teaspoon	Thyme
1 teaspoon	Rosemary
3 tablespoons	Fresh parsley, chopped
¾ teaspoon	Coarse Ground Black Pepper
¾ teaspoon	Salt
A dash	Chipotle chili powder
1 tablespoon	Butter or Ghee
1 tablespoon	Almond, coconut or tapioca flour
2 cups	Mushroom, Chicken or Vegetable broth

Directions:

1. In a large frying pan, heat 2 tablespoons of oil on medium-high heat. Add the onion, ¼ teaspoon salt and ¼ teaspoon pepper, stirring occasionally until onions brown. Remove and set aside.

2. Add remaining tablespoon of oil and raise heat to high. Add brown mushrooms, ¼ teaspoon salt and pepper, and chipotle. Cook for about 3 minutes, stirring constantly.

3. Reduce heat to medium, add herbs and tomato paste. Stir in tomatoes and cook for a minute or so. Dust with the flour, stirring to mix well and cook for another minute. Add cooked onions back in.

4. Add the broth and stir until thickened. Gradually add the second cup of broth, simmering for a few more minutes. This is a stew, so the sauce should be thick. You may thin it with more broth if desired. Keep warm.

5. Just before serving, add wild mushrooms to a separate frying pan with warmed and slightly browned butter, combined with 1 tablespoon oil on medium-high heat. Add remaining ¼ teaspoon of salt and pepper, garlic and parsley, coating the mushrooms with the mixture. Cook another minute then add to brown mushroom mixture. Serves 4 to 6.

Sausages in Tomato Sauce

Ingredients:

2 tablespoons	Butter or your desired fat
2 medium	Bell Peppers, cut into thin strips
1 medium	Onion, diced
12oz	Sausage of your choice, cut into small cubes
1 can (7oz)	Diced Tomatoes, drained
1 can (25oz)	Tomato Sauce
1 tablespoon	Apple Cider Vinegar
1 teaspoon	Garlic Powder
1 teaspoon	Dried Basil
1 pinch	Salt
1 pinch	Ground Black Pepper

Directions:

1. Melt fat in a large pot over medium heat.

2. Sauté onions and peppers until tender and mix in sausages. Cook for a few minutes.

3. Add diced tomatoes, tomato sauce, dried basil, garlic powder, apple cider vinegar, salt and pepper. Mix and partially cover.

4. Adjust heat to low and simmer for 20 minutes.

5. Serve with cooked rice or noodles, pasta or bread.

Frugal Stroganoff

Ingredients:

1 lb	Ground Beef
8 oz	White Mushrooms, sliced
1 large	Onion, diced
2 tablespoons	Ghee or Butter
2 tablespoons	Coconut Oil or Olive Oil
2 tablespoons	Tomato Paste
1 ½ teaspoons	Thyme
1 ½ teaspoon	Rosemary
4 cloves	Garlic, diced
1 tablespoon	Arrowroot Powder
1 ½ cup	Beef Stock
2/3 cup	Thick Coconut Cream (the cream on top of canned coconut milk)
½ teaspoon	Salt
½ teaspoon	Black Pepper, ground
	Cooked Zucchini Noodles

Directions:

1. Melt ghee or butter in a skillet with coconut oil or olive oil over medium heat.

2. Sauté onions and mushrooms until tender. Transfer to a plate and set aside.

3. In the same skillet, brown ground beef and stir in sautéed mushrooms.

4. Add garlic, thyme, rosemary and tomato paste.

5. Reduce heat to medium low and sprinkle arrowroot powder. Mix until arrowroot is completely combined in.

6. Pour in beef stock and mix. As the liquid thickens, reduce heat to low and simmer.

7. Turn off heat. Slowly add coconut cream and mix in.

8. Serve on top of cooked zucchini noodles.

"No Beans about It" Pumpkin Chili

Ingredients:

1 ½ lbs	Ground beef
1 ½ lbs	Ground turkey
2 cups	Red onion, diced
2 cups	Red and Green Bell Pepper
3 cloves	Garlic, peeled and minced
6 to 8	Tomatoes on the vine, diced with juice saved
3 cups	Pumpkin; cubed, boiled and mashed
6 ounces	Tomato paste
1 cup	Beef broth
2 tablespoons	Chili powder
1 ½ tablespoons	Dijon mustard
2 tablespoons	Coconut oil
1 ½ teaspoons	Coriander
½ teaspoon	Salt
½ teaspoon	Ground cinnamon
¼ cup	Cilantro, coarsely chopped

Directions:

1. In a large stew pot, heat oil on medium. Add onions and stir occasionally until brown. Throw in bell peppers and garlic, tossing them around in the pot for 5 minutes. Add 3 seeded and diced jalapeños for an additional spicy kick.

2. Combine beef and turkey, broth, tomatoes, tomato paste, mustard and spices into the pot with the onions and bell peppers and simmer for 20 to 25 minutes.

3. Mix pumpkin and cilantro in well, cooking for a few more minutes.

4. Serve hot or keep warm until ready. Great for leftovers, serves 8 to 10.

Pan-Fried Chicken with Steamed Vegetable Medley

Chicken Ingredients:

5 to 7 ounces	Organic Chicken Breast
1 tablespoon	Olive Oil
1 ½ tablespoons	Balsamic Vinegar
2 teaspoons	Apple Cider Vinegar
1/3 cup	Water
A sprinkling	Oregano
A dash	Coarse Ground Black Pepper
A pinch	Sea Salt
A sprinkling	Paprika
A sprinkling	Turmeric

Chicken Directions:

1. In a frying pan over medium heat, coat the surface with the olive oil. Make sure the pan is hot.

2. Put the chicken in the pan and brown it on both sides, sealing in the juices.

3. Reduce the heat to medium-low. Pour the balsamic and apple cider vinegars in over the chicken. Follow up by adding the water in the side of the pan. Cover quickly and let cook for 5 minutes.

4. Introduce the spices over the chicken breast then cover again. Increase the heat back to medium.

5. Cook until there is no pink in the thickest part of the breast by cutting it open and looking, or stick a meat thermometer into the thickest part of the breast and make sure it reaches 165° Fahrenheit. Remove from heat once done cooking.

Vegetable Medley Ingredients:

¼ large	Red or Yellow Onion, thinly sliced
¼ medium	Red Bell Pepper, sliced into lengthwise strips
¼ medium	Green Bell Pepper, sliced into lengthwise strips
¾ cup	Broccoli Florets, leave small ones whole and halve or quarter larger ones
¼ medium	Yellow Squash, thinly sliced
1 ½ tablespoons	Red Wine Vinegar

Vegetable Medley Directions:

1. In a medium-sized pot, add ½ to ¾ cup water and boil over medium heat.

2. Insert a steaming colander into the pot, and then add the vegetables and cover. Reduce to low heat and simmer for 3 minutes.

3. Remove the cover, pour in the red wine vinegar over the vegetables, then cover again and steam for an additional 4 to 5 minutes. The vegetables will be done when you stick a fork in the broccoli and it is soft.

4. Strain the vegetables. Season to taste with salt and/or pepper. Serve together with the chicken. Bon Appetite!

Leek Casserole

Ingredients:

2	Leeks
3	Carrots
1 head	Broccoli
3 medium to large	Potatoes
2	Cloves of Garlic, peeled
1 ½ teaspoons	Thyme
1 large	Onion
2 tablespoons	Olive Oil
3 cups	Vegetable broth
3 tablespoons	Cornstarch

Directions:

1. Cube and boil potatoes until semi-soft (do not overcook them!). Strain and rinse with cold water.

2. Preheat oven to 400° Fahrenheit

3. Chop all the vegetables and cook in a pan with the olive oil for 10 minutes or until brown, excluding the garlic, thyme and potatoes.

4. In a separate bowl, mix the vegetable broth and cornstarch well. Let sit.

5. Put cooked veggies and potatoes in a 9" x 11" glass baking dish. Mince the garlic and sprinkle on top, along with the thyme.

6. Pour the broth and cornstarch mix evenly over the vegetables

7. Bake the dish in the oven for 15 minutes. Remove from oven and let sit 5 to 10 minutes then serve.

Easy Pot Roast

Ingredients:

3 lb	Chuck Roast
2 tablespoons	Ghee
1 cup	Beef Stock
3 cloves	Garlic, minced
1	Onion, sliced
3 small	Carrots, chopped
1 teaspoon	Dried Oregano
2 teaspoons	Cumin
2 stalks	Celery, chopped
½ teaspoon	Paprika
1 pinch	Salt
1 pinch	Pepper

Directions:

1. Massage chuck roast with cumin, paprika, oregano, salt and pepper until well coated.

2. In a pan, melt ghee over medium heat and sauté onions until tender.

3. Stir in garlic, celery and carrots. Sauté until fragrant and soft.

4. Transfer into slow cooker.

5. In the same pan, melt remaining ghee and heat roast until all sides are brown. Transfer into slow cooker.

6. Pour in beef stock and slow cook for 6 to 8 hours.

7. You may add salt and pepper before serving to taste.

Swiss Steak

Ingredients:

2 lbs	Grass-fed Round Steak
4 tablespoons	Potato Starch, seasoned with salt and pepper
2 tablespoons	Butter or Ghee
1 medium	Onion, chopped
6 medium	Tomatoes, chopped
2 medium	Green Chilies
3 cloves	Garlic, minced
¼ cup	Red Wine
2 tablespoons	Liquid Aminos
1 cup	Water

Directions:

1. Cut steak into 6 slices.

2. Pound each side of the steak using the back of your knife or meat mallet to tenderize.

3. Coat meat lightly by dipping into seasoned potato starch.

4. Heat butter or ghee in a large skillet over medium heat. Fry steak slices and brown both sides. Transfer into crockpot.

5. In the same pan, sauté onions. Add more butter if needed. Transfer to crockpot.

6. Deglaze pan with wine and liquid aminos. Pour all tidbits from the pan into the crockpot including aminos and wine.

7. In a bowl, mix together garlic, water and tomatoes and pour over steak.

8. Cover crockpot and cook on low for 8 to 10 hours.

Chicken Artichoke

Ingredients:

2 tablespoons	Butter or Ghee
2 lbs	Chicken, sliced into lengthwise bite-size pieces
2 medium	Bell Peppers, cut into strips
9 hearts	Artichoke, rinsed and cut into quarters
2	Lemons, juiced
1 teaspoon	Dried Basil
1 pinch	Salt
1 pinch	Ground Black Pepper

Directions:

1. Melt butter or ghee in a large skillet over medium heat and cook chicken in it.

2. Season with salt and pepper. Feel free to add more fat if needed so it doesn't dry out.

3. When chicken is about to be done, add artichokes, bell pepper, lemon juice, dried basil, salt and pepper.

4. Mix until all vegetables are thoroughly cooked.

Citrus Chicken Marinade

Ingredients:

4	Boneless Chicken Breasts
1 cup	Freshly squeezed orange juice
2 tablespoons	Freshly squeezed lemon juice
½ teaspoon	Salt
½ teaspoon	Ground Black Pepper
2 cloves	Garlic, minced
4 sprigs	Fresh Thyme
1 handful	Chives, chopped (for garnish)

Directions:

1. Mix together lemon juice, orange juice, thyme, pepper and salt in a bowl.

2. Add in chicken breasts and make sure they are evenly coated with the mixture. Keep in the refrigerator and marinate for 4 to 8 hours.

3. Drain and pat chicken dry.

4. Brush grill pan with oil and place over medium heat.

5. Cook chicken until golden brown in each side. Slice thinly and garnish with chives.

Shrimp Stir-fry

Ingredients:

5 oz	Shrimp, peeled and deveined
1 large	Yellow Squash, chopped
1 large	Green Zucchini, chopped
1 medium	Red Bell Pepper, chopped
1 medium	Green Bell Pepper, chopped
1 large	Red Onion
4 stalks	Celery
6	Baby Eggplant
5 oz	Fresh Spinach Leaves
3 tablespoons	Sesame Oil
3 tablespoons	Coconut Aminos
½ teaspoon	Sea Salt (Himalayan)
½ teaspoon	Coarse Ground Black Pepper
¼ teaspoon	Cayenne (Red) Pepper
7	Cloves of Garlic, minced
2 ounces minced	Fresh Ginger Root, peeled and

Directions:

1. Note that due to the portion size, you may have to use two large saucepans to prepare this meal, or you can choose to halve the portions. Heat a large saucepan (or two) or a wok on medium-low for 1 minute. Add in sesame oil and heat, covering the surface of the pan(s) or wok.

2. Add in the garlic and ginger and cook for 1 – 1 ½ minutes.

3. Stir in all the vegetables, making sure that they are completely coated with oil. Cover and cook for 5 minutes, stirring occasionally.

4. Add in the spices and liquid aminos, stirring until the vegetables are coated evenly. Cover and cook for another 5 minutes or until vegetables have lost their crispiness yet are still mildly firm. Stick a fork or knife in the eggplant, bell peppers or celery and look for them to have some give.

5. Cut the shrimp into ½" sized portions and add into the pan. Cover and cook 3 – 5 minutes, watching carefully for the shrimp meat to turn an opaque white, letting you know that they are done. It does not take long for them to cook.

6. Serve and enjoy! Makes 8 to 10 servings.

Marinated Pork Chops

Ingredients:

4 – 8	Pork Chops, thick cut
4 cloves	Garlic, minced
1/3 cup	Honey
¼ cup	Red wine vinegar
¼ cup	Worcestershire Sauce
1 cup	Coconut aminos

Directions:

1. Mix all ingredients in a large zip lock bag, placing the pork chops in last.

2. Refrigerate at least 24 hours, turning the chops over every 4 hours.

3. Cook over a hot grill, 5 to 10 minutes on each side.

4. Serve.

Spiced Pineapple Pork Roast

Ingredients:

4 lbs	Pork Roast
12 ounces	Pineapple Preserves
2 tablespoons	Organic Honey
2 tablespoons	Red Wine Vinegar
1 teaspoon	Yellow Mustard
¼ teaspoon	Salt
¼ teaspoon	Cinnamon Powder
¼ teaspoon	Ground Cloves
8 ounces	Pineapple slices (rings)

Directions:

1. Put the roast on the oven rack in a shallow roasting pan. Stick a meat thermometer into the thickest part of the roast, avoiding touching any bones.

2. Roast the meat, uncovered, at 350° Fahrenheit for about 2 ½ to 3 hours or until the meat thermometer reaches 170°.

3. Combine the pineapple preserves, honey, vinegar, mustard, salt, cinnamon and cloves together in a small saucepan. Cook over low heat on the stove, stirring constantly, until the preserves melt.

4. At the last 20 minutes of roasting time, dress the pork roast with the pineapple slices and brush with the pineapple glaze several times using a basting brush.

5. Serve the leftover glaze with the warm roast. Makes about 6 servings.

Stuffed Cabbage

Stuffed Cabbage Ingredients:

1 large	Head of Cauliflower, cut lengthwise into 4 sections
1 ½ lbs	Ground Grass-fed Beef
1 large	Head of Green (or Red) Cabbage
¼ teaspoon	Salt
½ teaspoon	Paprika
½ teaspoon	Coarse Ground Black Pepper
1/8 teaspoon	Cayenne (Red) Pepper

Stuffed Cabbage Directions:

1. Use a cheese grater with medium-sized holes to grate the cauliflower sections into Paleo-friendly rice-sized bits.

2. Dry the excess juices from the cauliflower rice by placing them in a towel or paper towel and gently pressing down on them so that they do not cause the recipe to turn soggy. Set aside.

3. In a large saucepan over medium-low heat, brown and separate the ground beef into small bits. When it is done cooking, remove from heat and place in a large bowl.

4. Combine the cauliflower rice and spices together with the cooked meat, mixing well. Set aside.

5. Fill a large pot with water and submerge the cabbage head into it to make sure that it fits and is covered by the water, but not overflowing the pot. Cabbage floats, so you will have to press down on it.

6. Remove the cabbage from the pot and heat the water on high until it comes to a rolling boil.

7. Have a large plate and a pan cover for it ready next to the stove. Submerge the cabbage head upside-down in the pot so that the stalk is facing up. Boil until the outermost leaves become soft and begin to separate from the head. Use a carving fork to test for softness.

8. Once the outer leaves have softened, stick the carving fork into the cabbage stalk to hold it in place and cut the softened leaves free at the base. Place the free-cut leaves on the plate next to the stove and cover so that the heat is retained and the leaves do not stiffen.

9. Repeat steps 7 and 8 until you get to the core of the cabbage. The smallest leaves will not be used.

10. Preheat the oven to 350° Fahrenheit.

11. Set up a 9" x 13" baking pan or glass dish next to the stuffing and cabbage leaves. You will want to work at a good speed to prevent the cabbage from stiffening. Use a spoon to place 2 – 4 tablespoons of stuffing in the middle of a leaf.

12. Fold and roll the leaf up like a burrito by bringing the stem-end up and just over the pile of stuffing, tuck the sides of the leaf into the center so they are hugging the stuffing pile, and then roll tightly up to the top of the

leaf. Place the cabbage roll into the baking dish so that it sits on the top of the leaf.

13. Repeat steps 10 and 11 until you have run out of leaves or stuffing. Pack the baking dish tightly. If there is no more room, you can either stack the remaining rolls on top of the first layer or put them in a second baking dish. You may choose to use toothpicks, 1 for each roll stuck in the middle, to hold them together, but be sure to remove them before eating! If you roll well however, the cabbage should hold itself together without any problem.

14. Bake in the oven for 15 minutes.

Sauce Ingredients:

16 ounces	Tomato Sauce
2	Lemon Wedges
1 ½ tablespoons	Organic Honey

Sauce Directions:

1. Heat the tomato sauce in a large saucepan on medium-low to low heat, stirring occasionally.

2. Squeeze the lemons into the pan, minding that no seeds go in. Add in the honey and continue stirring.

3. You might like to change the portions of lemon and honey according to personal taste, going for a sweet-tangy flavor. Continue cooking until the sauce thickens.

4. At the last 5 minutes of baking, remove the cabbage rolls from the oven and drizzle the sauce over them, covering

them as much as possible. Put back in the oven for the remaining 5 minutes.

5. Serve warm with a spatula.

Sides, Soups and Salads

Glazed Carrots

Ingredients:

1 pound	Carrots; washed, peeled, stemmed and chopped in rounds
5 cups	Water
¼ cup (half stick)	Butter
1 to 2 tablespoons	Yellow mustard
1 tablespoon	Dried parsley flakes
1/3 cup	Honey

Directions:

1. Boil water in medium pot on medium-high heat. Add carrots and boil them to desired tenderness. Drain.

2. Leave carrots in pot on low heat. Melt butter in with them, then add other ingredients once melted.

3. Stir and serve.

Sautéed Onions

Ingredients:

1 cup	Leeks, chopped
1 cup	Onion, julienned
1 ounce	Fresh ginger, peeled and minced
2 to 3 cloves	Garlic, peeled and minced
1 ½ tablespoons	Honey
½ teaspoon	Coarse Ground Black Pepper
¼ teaspoon	Salt
1 tablespoon	Olive oil (or other desired oil)

Directions:

1. Heat oil in a frying pan on low.

2. Add ginger and garlic, cook stirring constantly for 30 seconds to 1 minute

3. Reduce heat to a simmer, add onions and leeks, then honey, salt and pepper.

4. Cover, stirring occasionally. Cook on simmer until onions caramelize, about 25 to 30 minutes.

5. Remove from heat and serve as a side to complement any meal.

Roasted Potatoes with Cilantro

Ingredients:

1 1/2 lb	Potatoes, washed and cut into cubes
1 large	Red Onion, cut into wedges
1 tablespoon	Olive Oil
1	Lemon, juiced (zest needed)
1 sprig	Fresh Cilantro, chopped
1 teaspoon	Garlic Powder
1 pinch	Salt
1 pinch	Ground Black Pepper

Directions:

1. Preheat your oven to 375°F.

2. In a bowl, mix together potatoes, onions, lemon zest, olive oil, cilantro, garlic powder, salt and pepper. Mix thoroughly until all potatoes are coated evenly.

3. Bake for 30 to 45 minutes or until onions and potatoes are thoroughly roasted.

4. Transfer in a salad bowl and spritz some lemon juice. Mix until well blended.

Butternut Squash Soup

Ingredients:

2 medium	Butternut Squash, cut into half and gutted
1 can	Coconut Milk
2 tablespoons	Coconut Oil
4 cups	Water
1 tablespoon	Ginger, ground
1 handful	Cilantro, chopped
2 teaspoons	Salt
2 teaspoons	Ground Pepper

Directions:

1. Preheat oven to 350° F.

2. If you want, you can roast the seeds you got from the butternut squash. Brush the flesh of the butternut squash with coconut oil.

3. Line your baking sheet with aluminum foil. Place butternut squash halves with the flesh side facing down. Roast until tender.

4. Remove from oven and cool until warm to touch.

5. Spoon out flesh and place in a large pot or Dutch oven.

6. Pour in water and coconut milk. Blend using a hand blender until creamy and smooth. You can use a conventional blender but puree in batches.

7. Stir in cilantro, ginger, pepper and salt. Mix until all lumps are dissolved.

8. You may add parmesan cheese of you like.

Gluten Free Tomato Soup

Ingredients:

2 tablespoons	Butter or Ghee
1 medium	Onion, diced
4 cloves	Garlic, diced
12oz	Sausages, sliced into bite-size cuts
2 cans (28oz)	Crushed Tomatoes
1 can (28oz)	Diced Tomatoes
1 cup	Coconut Milk or Heavy Cream
1 ½ cup	Chicken Stock
1 teaspoon	Garlic Powder
½ teaspoon	Cumin
1 ½ teaspoon	Dried Basil
2 tablespoons	Balsamic Vinegar
1 pinch	Salt
1 pinch	Ground Pepper

Directions:

1. In a large pot, melt butter or ghee over medium heat.

2. Sauté garlic and onions. Sprinkle with some salt.

3. Mix in sausages and cook until brown.

4. Add tomatoes (diced and crushed), coconut milk or heavy cream, chicken stock, balsamic vinegar, basil, cumin and garlic powder.

5. Lower heat and let simmer for 30 minutes. Season with salt and pepper.

6. Serve warm.

Onion Soup

Ingredients

4 large	White Onions, sliced
½ tablespoons	Balsamic Vinegar
1 tablespoon	Maple Syrup or Honey
4 cups	Chicken Stock
½ cup	Coconut Milk
2 tablespoons	Butter or Ghee
1 pinch	Salt
1 pinch	Ground Black Pepper

Directions:

1. In a saucepan, melt ghee or butter over medium heat.

2. Sauté onions until golden and soft.

3. Drizzle with vinegar and honey or maple syrup and stir vigorously.

4. Pour in chicken stock and bring to a boil. Lower down heat.

5. Remove from heat and puree using an immersion blender until smooth.

6. Simmer over low heat and add coconut milk. Season with salt and pepper.

Carrot Soup with Ginger and Zucchini

Ingredients:

8 medium	Carrots, peeled and chopped
2 medium	Zucchini, peeled and chopped
1 small	Onion, diced
1 medium	Apple, peeled and chopped
2 tablespoons	Ginger, minced
1 teaspoon	Turmeric
1 pinch	Cinnamon Powder
4 cups	Chicken Stock or Vegetable Stock
1 cup	Coconut Milk
2 tablespoons	Cooking fat (ghee, butter or lard)
1 pinch	Salt
1 pinch	Ground Black Pepper

Directions:

1. Melt your desired cooking fat in a saucepan over medium heat.

2. Sauté ginger and onion until soft and aromatic.

3. Stir in vegetables, apples and spices. Mix well and cook until carrots are tender.

4. Pour in stock and boil. Lower down heat to low and simmer.

5. Remove from heat and puree using an immersion blender.

6. Stir in coconut milk and simmer on low for a few minutes.

Mushroom Soup

Ingredients:

1 ½ lbs	Wild Mushrooms, sliced
2 large	Shallots, diced
1 tablespoon	Fresh Thyme, chopped
7 cups	Chicken Stock
1 cup	Coconut Milk
3 tablespoons	Ghee
¼ cup	Fresh Parsley, chopped
2 tablespoons	Tapioca Starch
1 pinch	Salt
1 pinch	Ground Black Pepper

Directions:

1. In a saucepan, heat ghee over medium temperature. Sauté shallots until tender.

2. Stir in mushrooms and thyme and cook until moisture starts to come out of the mushrooms.

3. Pour in chicken stock and boil over medium heat. Adjust heat to low and simmer for 15 minutes.

4. Slowly pour in coconut milk and season with salt and pepper. Mix slowly.

5. Add tapioca starch to thicken soup. Turn off heat and garnish with chopped parsley.

Tomato Carrot Soup

Ingredients:

4 large	Tomatoes, cored and halved
1 ½ cups	Carrots, shredded
1 cup	Fresh Spinach, chopped
1 small	Red Onion, chopped
3 cloves	Garlic, minced
¼ cup	Almond Milk (may substitute with coconut milk)
2 tablespoons	Olive Oil
1 pinch	Salt
1 pinch	Ground Black Pepper

Directions:

1. Preheat your oven to350°F.

2. In a baking sheet, arrange tomatoes, cut side facing down.

3. Roast in the oven for 15 to 20 minutes. Set aside to cool until warm enough to touch.

4. Peel off tomato skin and discard.

5. Heat olive oil in a saucepan over medium heat.

6. Sauté onion, garlic and carrots until tender.

7. Stir in peeled tomatoes and spinach until wilted.

8. Turn off heat and add almond milk. Puree using immersion blender.

9. Simmer over low heat and season with salt and pepper.

10. Serve while hot.

Summer Zest Soup

Ingredients:

8 – 14	Baby Red Potatoes with skins on, halved or cubed
3 medium	Onions (white or red), chopped
1 ½ cups	Frozen Spinach (or 3 cups fresh)
6 crushed	Vine Tomatoes
2	Golden Beets, cubed
2 large	Cloves of Garlic, peeled and minced
2 ounces	Ginger root, peeled and minced
¼ cup	Red Wine Vinegar
6 – 8 cups	Water
¼ teaspoon	Rosemary
¼ teaspoon	Thyme
½ teaspoon	Sweet Basil
1/8 teaspoon	Cinnamon powder
½ teaspoon	Salt
½ teaspoon	Black Pepper

Directions:

1. In a large pot, heat water on high until boiling. Add in potatoes and beets and continue boiling until they are semi-soft by sticking a fork or knife in them.

2. Reduce heat to medium-low and add the onions, tomatoes, garlic, ginger and red wine vinegar. Cook for 10 minutes.

3. Add in the spices and spinach. Reduce heat to low and cook an additional 5 to 10 minutes.

4. Serve.

Spicy Almond and Eggplant Soup

This is a beautiful, Paleo-friendly rendition of its peanutty cousin. It is great for warming up during the colder months, a lot like receiving a soothing hug from the inside. True to comparison, your body will be thanking you.

Ingredients:

1 lb	Eggplant, (peeled or not, your choice) and chopped
5 large	Shallots, peeled and thinly sliced
1 medium	Yellow Onion, diced
1	Hot Chili, seeded and minced
1/3 cup	Tomato Paste
2 cups	Tomatoes (with juice), diced
½ cup	Creamy Natural Almond Butter
½ lb	Green Beans, cut into 2" pieces
¼ cup	Almonds, sliced (optional)
5 cups	Water or Vegetable Broth
1" cube (1 ½ ounces)	Fresh Ginger, peeled and minced
1/3 cup	Cilantro, chopped coarsely and packed lightly in measuring cup
2 tablespoons	Fresh Squeezed Lemon Juice
5 tablespoons	Almond Oil

1 ½ teaspoons	Ground Cumin
1/8 to ¼ teaspoon	Cayenne (Red) Pepper (optional)
2 teaspoons	Ground Coriander
½ teaspoon	Turmeric
1 teaspoon	Salt

Directions:

1. Heat 2 tablespoons of almond oil in a large stew pot on medium-high heat. Add the shallots and fry, stirring occasionally, for about 20 minutes until browned and slightly caramelized. Remove the shallots and set them aside.

2. Add 2 more tablespoons of almond oil to the pot and then the eggplant, stirring to make sure the eggplant is completely coated. Cook for 12 to 15 minutes to a reasonable tenderness. Their color will become slightly translucent and lightly browned. Remove from heat and place in the same bowl as the shallots.

3. Add the remaining tablespoon of almond oil to the pot and toss in the onion, frying it until it becomes soft, translucent and slightly caramelized – about 5 minutes. Next add the ginger and chili pepper and cook for 1 minute. Following up, add in the cumin, salt, cayenne, coriander and turmeric and cook for an extra 30 seconds to 1 minute just so their smell becomes robust.

4. Toss in the tomatoes (save the juice for later!), stirring this mixture until it develops into a sauce-like consistency – about 1 to 2 minutes.

5. Now add in the tomato juice, paste, water or vegetable broth, green beans, as well as the cooked eggplant and shallots. Stir to combine well and on medium-high heat, bring to a boil for 5 minutes then reduce heat to simmer.

6. In order to blend the almond butter well with the soup, known as emulsification, put the almond butter in a separate bowl and add a ladleful of the soup broth to it. Stir until creamy and completely blended. Now add this mixture back into the pot, scraping every last bit of it in. Stir the soup to complete combining.

7. Cover and simmer on medium-low heat for 35 to 45 minutes, checking to see that the eggplant is very tender.

8. Remove the pot from the heat and stir in the lemon juice and cilantro.

9. Let cool for 15 to 30 minutes. When serving, you may choose to garnish the soup with almond slices and a bit more cilantro. Word to the wise, it tastes even better heated up the following day.

Lemon Fruit Salad

Ingredients:

6	Mandarin/Clementine Oranges, peeled and segmented
4 large	Apples, seeded and diced
4	Kiwi Fruits, peeled and diced
½ cup	Pomegranate Seeds
½ cup	Blueberries, washed and drained
4 tablespoons	Juice from freshly squeezed lemon
½ cup	Avocado Oil
2 teaspoons	Poppy Seeds

Directions:

1. In a large salad bowl, toss all fruits together.

2. In a separate bowl, whisk avocado oil, poppy seeds and lemon juice until emulsified.

3. Drizzle the dressing over the fruits and toss until everything is coated evenly.

4. Cool in the refrigerator for a few minutes before serving.

Broccoli Salad with Strawberries

Ingredients:

4 cups	Broccoli Florets
2 cups	Fresh Strawberries, cut into half
¼ cup	Almonds, sliced
¼ cup	Red Onion, julienned
½ cup	Mayonnaise, low fat
2 tablespoons	Juice from freshly squeezed lemon
1 tablespoon	Honey
1 tablespoon	Poppy Seeds

Directions:

1. In a deep bowl, whisk together mayonnaise, honey, lemon juice and poppy seeds until well blended.

2. In a salad bowl, combine broccoli florets, onion, strawberries and almonds.

3. Drizzle mayonnaise dressing all over salad and toss gently to coat evenly.

4. Refrigerate for a few minutes and serve cold.

Red and Green Salad

Ingredients:

2 large	Cucumbers, sliced into round thins
4 cups	Fresh Strawberries, sliced thinly
¼ cup	Raspberry Vinegar/Apple Cider Vinegar
1 teaspoon	Dry Ground Mustard
1 teaspoon	White Onion, minced
1 cup	Olive Oil
¼ cup	Honey
1 tablespoon	Poppy Seeds

Directions:

1. In a deep bowl, mix together vinegar, mustard, onion, olive oil, honey and poppy seeds.

2. In a salad bowl, combine strawberry and cucumber slices.

3. Drizzle with dressing and toss to coat all slices evenly. Serve

Waldorf Salad

Ingredients:

6	Red Delicious Apples, chopped in bite-size pieces with skin on
1 cup	Celery, chopped
1 cup	Pecans, coarsely chopped
½ to 1 cup	Mayonnaise

Directions:

1. Combine ingredients in a medium-sized bowl. Add mayo in last and a bit at a time, moisten to taste.

2. Serve at room temperature. Refrigerate to store.

Avocado Shrimp Salad

Ingredients:

2 lbs	Shrimp, steamed, peeled and deveined
2 medium	Avocados, peeled and cut into small cubes
2 tablespoons	Red Onion, diced
1 sprig	Fresh Parsley, chopped
¼ cup	Olive Oil
¼ cup	Balsamic Vinegar
½ teaspoon	Garlic Powder
1 teaspoon	Dijon Mustard
1 pinch	Salt
1 pinch	Ground Black Pepper

Directions:

1. In a mixing bowl, combine olive oil, vinegar, garlic powder, mustard, salt and pepper.

2. In a salad bowl, combine avocados, shrimps and onions.

3. Pour dressing all over the salad and toss until everything is evenly coated.

4. Garnish with chopped parsley. Serve.

Seasoned Egg Salad

Ingredients:

8 large	Eggs, hard-boiled and chopped
2 tablespoons	Fresh Chives, chopped
1/3 cup	Mayonnaise
½ cup	Red Bell Peppers, roasted and diced
½ teaspoon	Paprika
1 pinch	Salt
1 pinch	Ground Black Pepper

Directions:

1. In a bowl, mix all ingredients together except the mayonnaise.

2. Stir in mayonnaise until well blended.

3. Season with salt and pepper.

4. Refrigerate for 45 minutes to 1 hour before serving.

Wilted Ginger Spinach

Ingredients:

10 oz	Fresh Spinach leaves
1 ½ oz	Fresh Ginger root, peeled and minced
3	Cloves of garlic, peeled and minced
2 tablespoons	Sesame Oil
3 ½ tablespoons	Coconut Aminos

Directions:

1. In a large saucepan, turn heat on medium-low and add in sesame oil. Heat oil for a minute and coat the surface of the pan with it.

2. Add in ginger and garlic, stirring and frying for 1 minute.

3. Throw in spinach leaves. Reduce heat to low and cover pan. Cook for 2 - 3 minutes.

4. When volume of spinach leaves has reduced by half, pour in liquid aminos over entire surface. Cover and continue cooking on low for another two minutes.

5. Remove from heat and stir with a fork until spinach is completely coated and reduced in volume.

6. Serve as a snack or side dish.

Sautéed Beet Greens, Version 1

If you buy beets with the greens still intact, you may find yourself simply removing the greens and tossing them away. Here is a great recipe to make use of those greens that are still packed with healthy nutrients.

Ingredients:

4 cups	Beet Greens
2 stalks	Scallions (Green Onions), chopped
1 ½ teaspoons	Dijon Mustard
1 tablespoon	Horseradish
2 tablespoons	Olive Oil
¼ cup	Water

Directions:

1. Heat a large saucepan on medium-low, then add in the olive oil and cover the surface of the pan.

2. Add in the rest of the ingredients, stirring to coat everything evenly.

3. Cook the greens until they have wilted.

4. Add the water, cover the pan and simmer for about 2 − 3 minutes.

5. Serve as a snack or side dish.

Sautéed Beet Greens, Version 2

Ingredients:

4 cups	Beet Greens
2 stalks	Scallions (Green Onions), chopped
2 tablespoons	Garlic, peeled and minced
¼ teaspoon	Cayenne (Red) Pepper
1 pinch	Salt
1 pinch	Coarse Ground Black Pepper
2 tablespoons	Olive Oil
1 ½ tablespoons	Any Vinegar (Apple cider, Red wine, Balsamic, White, etc.)

Directions:

1. Heat a large saucepan on medium-low, add in the olive oil and coat the surface of the pan completely. Then add the garlic and cook for 1 minute

2. Add in the greens first, then the spices, stirring to cover them completely.

3. Cover the pan and cook 3 – 5 minutes.

4. Season with the vinegar.

5. Serve as a snack or side dish.

Bitterless Brussel Sprouts

Ingredients:

10 to 12	Brussel Sprouts, chopped
1 ounce	Fresh Ginger, peeled and minced
4	Cloves of Garlic, halved
1 ¼ tablespoons	Balsamic Vinegar
1 tablespoon	Apple Cider Vinegar
1 ½ tablespoons	Olive Oil
¼ teaspoon	Coarse Ground Black Pepper
¼ teaspoon	Salt

Directions:

1. In a frying pan over medium-low heat, cover the surface of the pan with the olive oil. Add the ginger and garlic, stirring and cooking them for 2 to 3 minutes to bring out their flavor.

2. Add the brussel sprouts and stir, making sure that they are completely coated. Cover, increase the heat to medium and cook for 2 to 3 minutes.

3. Introduce the balsamic and apple cider vinegars, followed by the salt and pepper. Reduce the heat back down to medium-low, stir well and cover. Cook for an additional 5 minutes or until brussel sprouts are tender.

4. Serve as a snack or side dish.

Stewed Apples

Ingredients:

8	Granny Smith apples; cored, peeled, and sliced into ½" thick pieces (approx. 8 slices per apple)
1/3 cup + 2 tablespoons	Honey
2 tablespoons	Ground Cinnamon

Directions:

1. In a large pot, add just enough water to cover the bottom (so the apples don't stick). Put the apples in with the honey and cinnamon. Stir to combine and coat.

2. Cook on medium heat, stirring occasionally, until apples are tender. Approximately 30 minutes cook time.

3. Serve as a side to warm roasts, beef and bird dishes.

Eggplant and Jicama Stir-fry

Ingredients:

½ large	Eggplant, cut into medium cubes, unpeeled
2 medium	Yellow squash, cut into medium chunks
1 large	Zucchini, cut into medium chunks
	Jicama, peeled and sliced into 1/8" chunks
2 large	Red onions, sliced
1 tablespoon	Balsamic vinegar
1 tablespoon	Coconut aminos
½ teaspoon	Coarse Ground Black Pepper
½ teaspoon	Salt
7 tablespoons	Olive or Coconut oil

Directions:

1. In a large frying pan, heat 3 tablespoons of oil on low. On low to warm heat, add onions, ¼ teaspoon of both salt and pepper to caramelize slowly for 45 minutes. Remove from pan and set aside.

2. Heat 3 more tablespoons of oil in the pan. Add the squash, zucchini and eggplant along with ¼ teaspoon

salt and pepper each. Stirring occasionally, cook on medium until brown and tender crisp.

3. Stirring constantly, add jicama and thrown the onions back in. Cook for about 3 minutes.

4. Add vinegar and aminos, stir to mix well.

5. Serve as a savory side to any main dish. Goes well with chicken or salmon.

Sweet Potato Casserole

Although it is quite delicious, if you are looking to lose weight then this recipe is not for you.

Casserole Ingredients:

3 cups	Sweet Potatoes, peeled and mashed (about 3 medium-sized raw sweet potatoes)
¾ cup	Organic Honey
2	Eggs, beaten
7 tablespoons	Coconut or Almond Milk
½ teaspoon	Salt
½ teaspoon	Pure Vanilla Extract

Casserole Directions:

1. Peel and cut the sweet potatoes into large chunks, about 1".

2. Place the sweet potatoes into a pot and fill it with water, just covering the top of them.

3. Boil the sweet potatoes on high heat until they have softened. Stick a fork or knife into them, looking for little to no resistance when doing so to know that they are done.

4. Strain. Place the sweet potatoes in a large bowl and mash them into a relatively even and smooth consistency.

5. Add in the rest of the ingredients and mix thoroughly.

6. Place the mixture into a 9" x 13" greased pan or glass dish (use grass-fed butter or olive oil to grease).

Topping Ingredients:

¾ cups	Organic honey
½ teaspoon	Aluminum-free Baking Soda
1 cup	Pecans, chopped
½ cup	Almond Flour
4 tablespoons (½ stick)	Grass-fed Butter

Topping Instructions:

1. Preheat the oven to 375° Fahrenheit.

2. Leave the butter out to soften slightly then cut up into small chunks. This will help it to mix more easily. Keep it somewhat solid; do not allow it to melt!

3. Mix all the ingredients together in a small to medium-sized bowl.

4. Spread the topping evenly over the sweet potato mixture in the dish.

5. Bake in the oven for 30 to 40 minutes, looking for the topping to turn golden to medium brown.

6. Serve, lick your lips and enjoy!

Accessory Recipes

Beef Bone Broth

(36 – 48 hrs. cook time; preferably need a slow cooker)

This recipe may appear to be involved but it is well worth the effort. Beef Bone Broth is one of the best things you can consume for the body, providing a hearty goodness for rich blood and bone marrow, healthy collagen, soft skin, and lubricated joints.

It is the ideal recipe for nursing sick people back to health rapidly. It can be eaten alone by anybody as a warm soup, or used as a beef bouillon base for other meals like stews. This recipe also yields about 12 to 14 cups, so you will have plenty of stock with versatility that will last you a long time.

Ingredients:

2	Beef Bones (about 5" – 6" long) (Desirably grass fed beef. If they are not, there will be foam on the surface when you slow cook them and you will have to skim the foam off).
2 ½ lbs	Oxtail Meat with Bones (found at your local butchery)
1 whole head	Garlic, separated and peeled
1 lb	Carrots, cut in 2" – 3" sections

1 whole bag	Celery (chop off bottom, then chop into big 2" – 3" sections, leaves and all. The reason for large chopped pieces is because any smaller and they will burn when roasting them.
2 large	Red onions, cut into large chunks
1 bag (10 oz)	Fresh Spinach Leaves
1 bunch	Kale, chopped
2 tablespoons	Apple Cider Vinegar
1 ½ teaspoons	Olive oil
1 tablespoon	Turmeric
About 12	Peppercorns
1 ½ teaspoons	Paprika
1/8 teaspoon	Cayenne (Red) Pepper
3	Bay Leaves
3 sprigs	Fresh Rosemary
3 sprigs	Fresh Thyme

Directions:

Prep:

1. Put the beef bones and oxtail in a large pot with enough water to cover the bones.

2. Add the apple cider vinegar.

3. Let them sit in the pot of water for 30 minutes. Save the pot of water once you remove the bones. The apple cider vinegar leeches out some of the nutrients of the bones and comes in use later.

Roasting:

1. Preheat the oven to 400° Fahrenheit.

2. On a large cooking sheet, lightly oil the bottom with extra virgin cold pressed olive oil then spread the vegetables, beef bones and oxtail on it.

3. Place the baking sheet in the oven and roast the vegetables, bones and oxtail for 20 minutes.

4. Take the sheet out of the oven and use tongs to rotate the bones and oxtail (upside-down) and turn and mix the vegetables. Add the garlic cloves anywhere onto the pan at this time (it must be done at this time otherwise they will burn).

5. Put the baking sheet back in the oven for another 20 minutes.

6. Repeat rotation and roasting for a third set of 20 min one more time (1 hour total).

Cooking:

1. While roasting the meat & vegetables, cover and cook down the kale and spinach in the pot of water that the bones were soaked in until they are soft and mushy (about 20 min boiling). You may need to add a bit more water to make sure that the kale and spinach are completely submerged.

Slow Cooker:

1. Turn the slow cooker on low.

2. Use tongs to place the bones and oxtail in the bottom of the slow cooker (do not add the grease from the meat left on the baking sheet).

3. Put the roasted vegetables on top of the bones, then scoop out the spinach and kale from the water and add them on top of that.

4. Add the water the spinach and kale cooked in to the top of the slow cooker (you won't use it all yet).

5. Add in the spices, peppercorns and herbs. Make sure to fully submerge the sprigs of rosemary and thyme. Cover the slow cooker.

6. Watch the slow cooker every couple of hours. Whenever you see that the level of the broth has dropped some (1/2 inch or less), continually add the remaining water that the spinach and kale cooked in to top off the slow cooker over the next 48 hours. You will notice the level of the broth drop over time, so just add in more water to level it off at the top. If you run out of the spinach/kale water, use faucet water.

Rendering:

1. After 48 hrs. of cooking, use tongs to remove the oxtail and discard it.

2. Take the beef bones out. Use a long, skinny knife or some other useful utensil to push all of the marrow in

the center of the bones out into a small container. Save this marrow and refrigerate it, then discard the bones.

3. Place the broth in the fridge to cool and render overnight.

4. After rendering, the fat that has formed a layer at the top of the broth can be scraped off and thrown away.

5. Add the marrow you saved back into the broth.

6. Take the bottom of a ladle to smash the marrow, as well as the veg, through the colander into the bowl, which you then will place back into the broth after it's been rendered. Discard what does not come through.

Jarring and Nutrient Extraction:

1. You will need about 6 – 7 jars with lids that hold 2 cups each to store the broth.

2. It might be a good idea to put paper towels or a cloth towel under each jar as you fill them in case of spillage.

3. Using a fine mesh colander and a ladle, place the colander over a jar and *very slowly and carefully*, ladle the broth into the jar. You will notice the vegetable and marrow remnants caught by the colander. Again, *slowly and carefully* use the bottom of the ladle to smash these vegetables through the colander to extract the nutrients that they contain. There will still be remnants in the colander that you can choose to then add to the jar or discard, depending on the viscosity of the broth that you prefer.

4. Repeat this process until every jar is full. Take note that some pieces of bone from the oxtail might still be in the broth, so be careful to check for them throughout this process.

Storage:

1. If you choose to freeze the jars and just pull them out when necessary, you need only clean them with soap and water before filling them. Shelf life = 8 to 12 months.

2. If you choose to store the jars in the fridge or pantry, you will need to boil them in a specialized pot for 20 minutes before filling them. This is called a sanitization pot and comes equipped with a special metal rack insert so that the glass jars do not break by sitting on the metal of the hot pot. Shelf life = 2 to 8 weeks.

Avocado and Coconut Milk Salad Dressing

Ingredients:

1/3 cup	Balsamic Vinegar
2/3 cup	Olive Oil
1/3 cup	Coconut Milk
2 tablespoons	Dijon Mustard
4 whole	Cloves of Garlic, peeled
½	Avocado
1 ½ teaspoons	Salt

Directions:

1. Put all ingredients in a blender, adding liquids first before solids so as not to block the blades.

2. Blend on the frappe setting until mixture is smooth.

3. Serve 1 to 2 tablespoons over any salad and enjoy! Refrigerate in a covered and sealed container to store.

Mexican Salsa

Ingredients:

1	Avocado, diced into small cubes
1 medium	Yellow Onion, diced
1 medium	Tomato, diced into small cubes
1	Lime wedge
¼ teaspoon	Salt

Directions:

1. Combine all ingredients into a small or medium-sized bowl, mixing well. Squeeze the lime over the top, removing any seeds beforehand.

2. Eat with a spoon as a small snack, as a side dish, or serve over a chicken breast or steak cut for a fresh twist.

Cardiovascular Cleanser

This recipe is great for removing LDLs (bad cholesterol) and tar (if you are a smoker or live in an area with high air pollution) from your arteries, veins and capillaries. No to mention it is packed with anti-inflammatory, antioxidant and other highly beneficial properties.

Ingredients:

1 ounce	Fresh ginger, peeled and grated (perforated side of grater)
2 cloves	Garlic, peeled and grated (perforated side)
1 tablespoon	Honey
1 large	Lemon, juiced and seeded
1 ½ cups	Water

Directions:

1. Save the juice from the prepped ginger and garlic, add in with other ingredients

2. Combine all ingredients into a blender or food processor and blend on high for 1 to 2 minutes.

3. Pour into a glass, scraping any leftover bits in as well. Drink to your health!

Sinus and Lymph Tonic

Ingredients:

1 tablespoon	Apple cider vinegar
1 to 2 cloves	Garlic, peeled and grated (on perforated side) with juice
1 ounce	Fresh ginger, peeled and grated (on perforated side) with juice
A small pinch	Cayenne (red) pepper
A dash	Coarse Ground black pepper
A pinch	Paprika
1 large	Lemon, seeded and juiced

Directions:

1. Combine all ingredients together in a small bowl, blender, food processor or straight in a cup

2. Pour tonic into a cup and swill to clean the sinus and lymph systems

Mama's Chock-full Smoothie

Ingredients:

1 cup	Coconut milk
2 tablespoons	Chia seeds
1 cup	Berries of choice (fresh or frozen)
1 cup	Spinach (fresh or frozen)
½	Lemon; zested, seeded and juiced
2 to 3 teaspoons	Ground cinnamon

Directions:

1. Combine all ingredients (including lemon zest) in a blender and blend until texture is smooth. Add chia seeds in last of ingredients so they don't get stuck at the bottom of the blender.

2. Add extra coconut milk or water if mixture is too thick.

Golden Milk

This is an ancient Ayurvedic drink, great before bedtime when the body is preparing to restore and regenerate itself. It has a smooth, slightly nutty taste.

You will want to prepare a reserve of Golden Paste so that you can just add a dollop to making the milk for quick preparation anytime of the day.

Golden Paste Ingredients:

½ cup	Turmeric powder
1 cup	Water
1 ½ teaspoons	Coarse ground black pepper
5 tablespoons	First-pressed Organic Virgin Coconut oil

Directions:

1. Heat the water in a pot on medium. Do not allow it to boil or it will destroy the nutrients of the turmeric and black pepper. Add these ingredients and stir consistently until the mixture forms a thick paste, about 8 minutes.

2. Remove pot from heat and whisk coconut oil in vigorously to blend well.

3. Store in a tight-lidded container and refrigerate. Lasts about 2 weeks.

Golden Milk Ingredients:

1 teaspoon	Golden paste
2 cups	Coconut milk (or almond milk)
A sprinkle	Cinnamon

Directions:

1. In a pot over medium-low heat, heat but do not boil the milk and paste, whisking them together.

2. Pour into a cup. Add cinnamon and honey as desired.

Chapter 6:
Your Shopping List

To maximize your Paleo experience, you should have your shopping list before going to the grocery. It will save you unnecessary trips to the store, save you more money and allow you to stock on foods that you will need for the coming days.

To keep fruits and vegetables fresh, it is recommended to buy your ingredients for a week. Stocking on fruits and vegetables for more than a week can compromise their quality and freshness even if you keep them refrigerated.

Before you list down the things you need to buy from the grocery store, you need to plan the meals that you will be preparing for the entire week. You can choose from the various meals listed in this book. To maximize your time, you can prepare some of your meals beforehand and keep them refrigerated. You may reheat them if necessary.

Sample shopping list for a week:

Meat

3 lbs	Ground Beef
1 tray	Large Eggs, about 30 pieces
2 ½ lbs	Shrimps

Vegetables

2 large	Spaghetti Squash
4 medium	Zucchini

1 bag	Spinach
2 heads	Romaine Lettuce
2 heads	Broccoli
2 lbs	Mushrooms
1 kilo	Bell Peppers
2 lbs	Tomatoes
1 lb	Onions
½ lb	Garlic
2 oz	Chives
2 oz	Parsley
2 oz	Celery

Fruits

½ kilo	Strawberries
4 large	Avocados
½ kilo	Kiwi
6 large	Apples
8 large	Pears
1 kilo	Grapes
3 large	Pomegranate

1 kilo	Mandarin/Oranges
4	Lemons
4 large	Cucumbers
½ lb	Blueberries

Seasonings/Spices

½ kilo	Salt
½ kilo	Black Pepper
1 pack	Ground Cinnamon
1 pack	Paprika
1 pack	Poppy Seeds
1 small bottle	Apple Cider Vinegar/Balsamic Vinegar
1 bottle	Olive Oil
1 medium bottle	Mayonnaise
1 pack	Ghee/Butter
2 cans	Coconut Milk/ Almond Milk
1 small bottle	Mustard
1 large bottle	Honey/Maple Syrup

As much as possible, choose recipes that have similar ingredients so you can stock up efficiently and practically. You would also notice that the seasonings/spices are too much for a week. That is okay because you can still use them in the next coming weeks or even months, as they stay fresh longer.

You make a shopping list to ensure that you have enough food for a week and to not waste food. Food is important and it must be treated with respect. In Paleo, you do not only learn which food is best for you, you also learn to value them.

Remember that this is only a sample shopping list. Yours should depend on what you need and what you can consume. Your budget is also a great factor. If you are near local stores and farmer's markets, better buy from them than from grocery stores. Also, choose fruits and vegetables that are in season as they are cheaper. You can always adjust your recipes according to what you have.

Chapter 7:
Your Paleo Checklist

As a beginner, you can't help but wonder if you are doing it right. Below is the checklist to help you figure out if you are doing it right and pinpoint your mistakes. This checklist is geared towards beginners to help them know what to and what not to do.

1. Your diet should be high in fats, contain moderate animal protein and low to medium carbohydrates. You should not be calorie counting nor should you be doing portion control. Paleo Diet is about eating healthy, not restricting yourself from eating. Counting your calories can be stressful and can lead to binge-eating in the end.

2. Eat a generous amount of saturated fats like butter or coconut oil. Animal fats such as beef tallow, duck fat or lard are also good as long as they originate from grass-fed animals. Olive oil, macadamia oil and avocado oil are also healthy fats you can use for your salads. These oils are not meant to be heated in high temperatures. Doing so can alter their natural composition and may have harmful effects.

3. Eat adequate amounts of animal protein in the form of meat, poultry, fish, sea foods, egg, organs, etc. So long as they are grass-fed, you should not be scared to eat the fatty cuts. Make use of the bones by turning them into stocks or broths. These are great for soups and meat dishes.

4. Eat a generous amount of vegetables (fresh or frozen). You can eat them in a form of salad (raw) or cooked with your favorite dishes. Vegetables should make up at

least 80% of your diet. You should have vegetables in every meal.

5. Eat fruits and nuts for snacks. Choose fruits that low in sugar and highly antioxidant like berries. Nuts that contain Omega 3 and low in polyunsaturated fats like macadamia are great for snacks. If you have an autoimmune disease, digestive issues or if you are trying to lose weight, refrain from eating nuts and sugary fruits.

6. Choose grass-fed or pasture-raised animals from your local farmer's market. If it's not possible, choose lean meats and supplement with coconut oil or butter. Organic fruits and vegetables are preferred. If you can't get one, choose the freshest from your grocery store and make sure to soak them in a basin of water mixed with 1 to 2 tablespoons of vinegar to help remove the chemicals and pesticides used by commercial manufacturers.

7. Stop from eating legumes or cereal grains. Wheat, oats, barley, brown rice, corn, peanuts, soy, beans and peas should be removed from your diet.

8. Hydrogenated or partly hydrogenated oils are not allowed. Olive oil and avocado oil should only be used for salads, do not cook with them. Use coconut oil or butter for cooking.

9. Dairy products should be excluded from your diet, but, if you can't live without them, you can use alternatives such as almond milk or coconut milk.

10. Refrain from eating anything that has added sugars such as soda, pastries or fruit juices.

11. Do not skip meals. Eat when you are hungry and learn to stop when you are full. Don't worry is you skip a meal or two, as long as you do not feel hungry. Listen to your body.

12. Getting enough sleep a day is important. Sleep at least 8 hours a day.

13. Exercise is good but do not overdo it. Choose short but intense training sessions instead of long cardio sessions.

14. Eat vegetables every day. When you work out, eat starchy vegetables for more carbs.

15. Enjoy your experience. Do not suppress your appetite. Paleo food is less dense compared to junk foods so you need to consume more so your body can get enough energy.

If you are not doing some of the statements above, chances are, you are depriving yourself of food, you are not consuming enough fats and your carbohydrates intake is inadequate.

If this is the case, don't feel bad. These are the common mistakes that beginners do. To ensure you get it right, stick to raw, organic fruits and vegetables and grass-fed or pasture-raised animals. If it's not possible, choose food products that have only 2 to 3 ingredients. If it's more than that, it's not good for you.

Do not be afraid to eat when you are hungry. Eating is good, what is bad is your food choices. When you are full, stop eating. If you still have some food left, store them in the refrigerator so you can eat them again later.

Conclusion

Thank you for reading this eBook.

The Paleo Diet is one of the most versatile and effective diet known to man. If you look at it closely it is not just a simple diet, it is a lifestyle. It basically requires you to go natural and choose what is best for your body.

Just like our ancestors before, they eat what was provided to them by nature. They rely on nature to keep them nourished. In this modern day, man are focused on making everything easy, instant, and likeable to the point of altering food to make them cheaper and marketable.

Paleo Diet gives your body a reset, helping you get rid of the deadly toxins that built up in your system. Since the toxins are released, your body systems will start to work optimally and your immune system will be enhanced. As an end result, you feel more energized, healthier, and emotionally stable.

You are what you eat, so it is important that you choose what you put inside your body. When your body organs are working well, your overall health is better, making you stronger, happier, and more productive.

If you enjoyed this book, please take the time to share your thoughts and post a positive review on Amazon. It'd be greatly appreciated!

Thank you and good luck!

To Leave A 5 Star Review - Click Here

Free Bonus + Subscription Link – Click Here

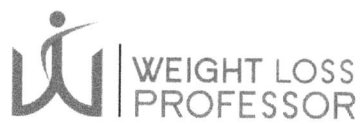
WEIGHT LOSS PROFESSOR

CPSIA information can be obtained
at www.ICGtesting.com
Printed in the USA
LVHW031230131218
600169LV00015B/416/P

9 781535 468930